To:

_____

From:

_____

Date:

_____

# Expecting

Praying for
Your Child's
Development—
Body and Soul

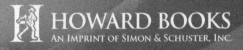

**HOWARD BOOKS**
AN IMPRINT OF SIMON & SCHUSTER, INC.

New York   London   Toronto   Sydney   New Delhi

Marla Taviano

Howard Books
An Imprint of Simon & Schuster, Inc.
1230 Avenue of the Americas
New York, NY 10020

Copyright © 2009 by Marla Taviano

First Howard Books trade paperback edition March 2016

HOWARD and colophon are trademarks of Simon & Schuster, Inc.

For information about special discounts for bulk purchases, please contact Simon & Schuster Special Sales at 1-866-506-1949 or business@simonandschuster.com.

The Simon & Schuster Speakers Bureau can bring authors to your live event. For more information or to book an event, contact the Simon & Schuster Speakers Bureau at 1-866-248-3049 or visit our website at www.simonspeakers.com.

Interior design by Tennille Paden
Illustrations by Katherine Cody Kicklighter

Manufactured in the United States of America

10  9  8  7  6  5  4  3  2  1

The Library of Congress has cataloged the hardcover edition as follows:

Taviano, Marla, 1975–
  Expectant prayers : praying for your child's development—body and soul / Marla Taviano.
      p. cm.
1. Pregnant women—Prayers and devotions. 2. Mothers—Prayers and devotions. 3. Fetus—Growth. 4. Fetus—Religious aspects—Christianity. I. Title.
  BV4847.T34 2009
  242'.6431—dc22
2008021156

ISBN 978-1-4165-7200-8
ISBN 978-1-5011-3987-1 (pbk)
ISBN 978-1-4767-3713-3 (ebook)

# Contents

# WEEK 1
## Prayer ∽ Uterine Lining

Before I formed you in the womb
I knew you, before you were born
I set you apart.

*Jeremiah 1:5a*

*Certainly the world owes more to the prayers
of women than it realizes.*

Herbert Lockyer

# A Prayer for Baby—Body and Soul

God, I know it's never too early to pray for my future children. Thoughts of motherhood have always had a place in my mind and heart. I'm not naïve enough to think it will be easy, but I know I can do this with you by my side.

God, will you watch over my body as it prepares to welcome a child into my womb? Will you work out everything for good and make sure the conditions are just right for conception?

I want to start praying even now for the child who will someday rest in my arms. Would you protect that baby? Would you help him grow up to be healthy and happy? To be a child who falls in love with Jesus and never stops growing in his relationship with you?

Please give me the discipline to pray for my child every day for the rest of my life.

In Jesus' name, Amen.

Before I formed you in the womb I knew you, before you were born I set you apart. —Jeremiah 1:5a

# Baby's Physical Development

No baby yet at this point. His parts are still nestled safely in two different bodies—Mom's and Dad's. It's amazing to think that a tiny egg (present in a woman's body since before she was born) can unite with an even tinier sperm from her partner's body and create a brand-new human being. Your uterine lining goes so baby can come!

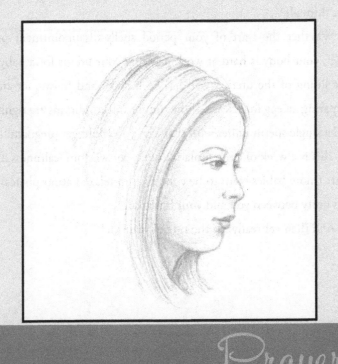

Prayer

# Mom's Development—Body and Soul

Oddly enough, the forty weeks of pregnancy start two weeks before your baby is even conceived. If you've been trying for a while, you're probably spending a lot of time talking to God about this desire of your heart. He's listening to those prayers!

If a baby wasn't in your plans right now, God knows this too. And He'll be there for you throughout your pregnancy, guiding you through.

Whether the start of your period spells disappointment or relief, your body is hard at work readying your uterus for a baby. The lining of the uterine wall has been shed, and hormones are preparing an egg for release. If the timing and conditions are right, and a single sperm unites with that egg, you could get pregnant!

This is a week of contemplation. Pray for wisdom, calmness of heart (more babies seem to be conceived in relaxed atmospheres), and unity between you and your husband.

And then get ready for the ride of your life!

*Before I formed you in the womb I knew you, before you were born I set you apart.* —Jeremiah 1:5a

# In Your Words

What one request is weighing on your heart right now? Write a prayer to God that addresses that need.

_____

_____

_____

_____

_____

_____

_____

_____

_____

_____

_____

_____

_____

_____

_____

_____

_____

_____

# WEEK 2

## Peace ∽ A Tiny Egg

Do not be anxious about anything, but
in everything, by prayer and petition, with
thanksgiving, present your requests to God.
And the peace of God, which transcends
all understanding, will guard your hearts
and your minds in Christ Jesus.

PHILIPPIANS 4:6–7

As a mother, my job is to take care of what is possible
and trust God with the impossible.

Ruth Bell Graham

# Mom's Development—Body and Soul

If you've been planning and praying for a baby, you're probably getting pretty anxious right now. You might find it hard to concentrate on anything but conceiving a child. It won't be long before you're ovulating and your body is at its most fertile time of the month.

In a perfect world, anticipation and excitement would precede every pregnancy, but it doesn't always work out that way. God can take an unsettling situation and unplanned pregnancy and turn it into one of life's biggest blessings.

You'll get used to this odd way of counting weeks of pregnancy. You've already started week 2! Soon you'll be happy to tack on two weeks to the age of your growing fetus when people ask, "How far along are you?"

Open your Bible this week and look for verses that speak about peace (and maybe patience). You'll appreciate them even more in the weeks and months to come.

# A Prayer for Baby—Body and Soul

Father, we're getting ever closer to the day that our little baby is a living, growing reality inside of me. It's so hard for me to wrap my mind around that possibility. There might be a baby in my near future! So many emotions are swirling around in my head.

I need your peace, God. I need you to wrap me in your arms and tell me everything is going to be okay. I need your blessed reassurance.

I don't know how you're going to calm my tangled-up emotions, but I believe you can. Your peace transcends my human understanding, but that's why you're God and I'm not.

Enough about me, Lord. I pray for my soon-to-be child. I so want her to get off to a beautiful start in life. I want her to be strong and independent and unique and glowing. I want her to know love and hope and faith. I want her to be everything she dreams of being—everything *you* dream for her.

*In Jesus' name, Amen.*

*Before I formed you in the womb I knew you, before you were born I set you apart. —Jeremiah 1:5a*

# Baby's Physical Development

Your baby is still just a thought in the mind of her parents. Only her Creator knows exactly when she will be conceived. Her mother's egg prepares for release, bringing with it Mama's characteristics to pass on to Baby. Likewise, the tiny sperm that wins the race to the egg brings attributes of Daddy's that will become a part of who she is.

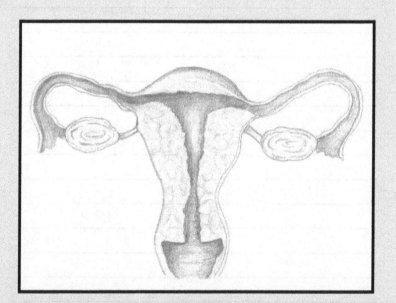

# In Your Words

Which verses about peace struck a chord in your heart and why?

_____

_____

_____

_____

_____

_____

_____

_____

_____

_____

_____

_____

_____

_____

_____

_____

_____

*Before I formed you in the womb I knew you, before you were born I set you apart. —Jeremiah 1:5a*

# WEEK 3

# New Divisions ∽ Conception

My frame was not hidden from you when
I was made in the secret place. When
I was woven together in the depths of the
earth, your eyes saw my unformed body.
All the days ordained for me were written
in your book before one of them came to be.

*PSALM 139:15–16*

*When you are a mother, you are never
really alone in your thoughts.
A mother always has to think twice,
once for herself and once for her child.*

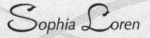

Sophia Loren

# A Prayer for Baby—Body and Soul

Father, my baby is here! He exists! I believe with all my heart that life begins at conception, and my child has been conceived! I can hardly wrap my mind around it.

I know scientists call it a zygote, nothing more than a bunch of cells dividing again and again, but I know I have a miracle inside my body. A baby! Part of his daddy, part of me. And in nine short months, I'll hold him in my arms.

I praise you for the mystery and miracle of life!

As my baby's cells divide, I can't help but think of the other kinds of dividing he'll do someday. He'll have to divide truth from lies. He'll need to divide his time among his many responsibilities. And someday, he'll divide—break away—from his daddy and me and cleave to his spouse.

God, please bless my child with discernment and wisdom. May he know the difference between good and evil, truth and falsehood. And may he never be separated—divided—from your love.

In Jesus' name, Amen.

Before I formed you in the womb I knew you, before you were born I set you apart. —Jeremiah 1:5a

# Baby's Physical Development

The egg and sperm have met in your fallopian tube. Your baby has been conceived! The head of the sperm and the nucleus of the egg unite to form a new cell—a zygote. The journey to your uterus takes seven to ten days. Then it implants in the uterine wall, and cells will begin to divide immediately.

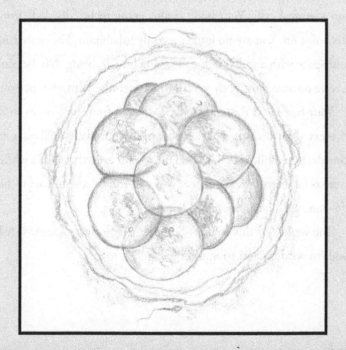

New Divisions

# Mom's Development—Body and Soul

You have ovulated, and one lucky sperm has penetrated your egg. Wow! When the fertilized egg implants, you might experience some spotting. Never fear—implantation bleeding is normal and results from the egg burrowing into your uterine lining.

The fertilized egg, called a zygote, immediately begins dividing into identical cells. Your body is also going to be "divided" from this point on. You are no longer its only inhabitant. You're sharing your space with another living, growing human being. No, he can't survive outside your body yet, but he is definitely his own person.

Your heart and thoughts will be divided from now on as well. In every decision you make, each action you take, you'll have to consider your child. He'll depend on you for everything for a while. Even as he gains independence, you will still be a vital part of his life—and he'll be an inextricable part of yours.

The weight of this responsibility isn't light by any means. Ask God for wisdom and strength. He'll give it to you.

*Before I formed you in the womb I knew you, before you were born I set you apart.* —Jeremiah 1:5a

# In Your Words

It's impossible to predict, of course, but in what ways do you see your life changing once you become a mommy?

_____

_____

_____

_____

_____

_____

_____

_____

_____

_____

_____

_____

_____

_____

_____

_____

_____

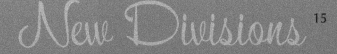

New Divisions

## Home ∽ Implantation

These commandments that I give you today
are to be upon your hearts. Impress them on
your children. Talk about them when you sit
at home and when you walk along the road,
when you lie down and when you get up.

*DEUTERONOMY 6:6–7*

*Home, the spot of earth supremely blest,*
*A dearer, sweeter spot than all the rest.*

Robert Montgomery

# Mom's Development—Body and Soul

So, you've seen that magical line on the pregnancy test. Or maybe yours was a plus sign, or even the words, "You're pregnant."

If you've been hoping and praying for a baby, you were thrilled to your toenails with the results on that little stick. Did your jaw drop? Did you squeal? Cry? Jump up and down?

If this pregnancy wasn't planned, you might be shocked, worried, or even scared. You'll need some time to process the news. And that's okay.

As the zygote nestles into your uterus and the gestational sac becomes her temporary home, take a moment to think about your own home—the place that will be home to your child once she leaves your womb and the hospital.

Home is more than four walls and a roof, more than your furniture and wall décor. Home is where the heart is, a place to relax and have fun, a place you long to return to after time away.

Think of ways you can make your home a warm and inviting place for your child to live and grow in. What can you do to help her childhood home be the kind of place that always stirs up fond memories of love and faith and laughter?

Home

# A Prayer for Baby—Body and Soul

Lord, right now my baby's home is a gestational sac that will help cushion and protect her in the months to come. She's in the safest place she can be, and I thank you for your perfect design that helps ensure her survival and comfort.

Will you help me make our home a safe haven too? I want my child to always feel like she can be herself, let her hair down in our home. I want her to feel like Mom and Dad are her biggest allies, that we would give ourselves to guarantee her safety and security.

May our home be the place she runs to when she needs shelter from the storms of life. May our home be a place she feels comfortable bringing her friends. May our home be a place where she learns about Jesus and feels his presence.

I'm so thankful that my child will begin her life in a home with a family. If only every child were so blessed.

In Jesus' name, I pray. Amen.

*Before I formed you in the womb I knew you, before you were born I set you apart. —Jeremiah 1:5a*

# Baby's Physical Development

Once the fertilized egg implants, it is called a blastocyst. The blastocyst divides into two parts—one part forms the placenta, and the other is your baby. The chorionic villi (part of the border between your blood and Baby's while you're pregnant) are fully formed at week's end. And the yolk sac (which feeds your baby until the placenta takes over) is starting to appear.

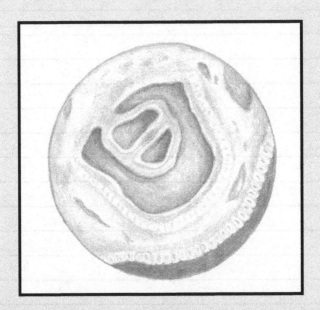

# In Your Words

What do you remember about the atmosphere of your childhood home(s)? Which parts would you like to re-create for your own children?

_____

_____

_____

_____

_____

_____

_____

_____

_____

_____

_____

_____

_____

_____

_____

_____

_____

*Before I formed you in the womb I knew you, before you were born I set you apart.* —Jeremiah 1:5a

# WEEK 5

## Intelligence & Brain

> Love the Lord your God with all your
> heart and with all your soul and with all
> your mind and with all your strength.
>
> MARK 12:30

*The human brain is a most unusual instrument*
*of elegant and as yet unknown capacity.*

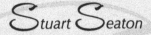

Stuart Seaton

# A Prayer for Baby—Body and Soul

Lord, I've barely had time to process that I'm pregnant, and my baby's tiny brain is already forming and developing. Such a miracle. What a complex organ the human brain is. I can't hope to ever understand it completely, but I take comfort in the fact that you designed it and know it inside and out.

I pray that you will bless my child with a fully functioning brain. May every cell and every lobe work precisely the way you designed it to work. May he constantly be learning and making new connections. I pray that I might do my part to make his environment conducive to intellectual stimulation and growth. His IQ doesn't matter, as long as he makes the most of what you've given him.

Father, help him to use his mind in hundreds of positive ways. Bless him with intelligence so that he might use it to be a blessing to others. Help him to love you, Lord, not just with his heart but with his mind.

In Jesus' name, Amen.

Before I formed you in the womb I knew you, before you were born I set you apart. —Jeremiah 1:5a

# Baby's Physical Development

Your miniature baby is about the size of a sesame seed and resembles a tadpole at this point. He's made up of three layers—the ectoderm, mesoderm, and endoderm. Soon these layers will form his vital organs and tissues. The neural tube is starting to develop in the top layer, the ectoderm. In other words, your baby's brain is already beginning to form!

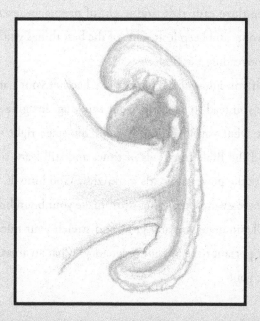

# Mom's Development—Body and Soul

You might not notice any changes in your body yet. Pregnancy symptoms coming soon!

As your baby's brain begins to develop, yours might seem to be missing a few cells. It's common for pregnant women to be forgetful. Don't worry—you're still the intelligent woman you've always been!

During these early days and weeks of pregnancy, exercise that mind of yours and keep it fit. One of the best things you can do is spend time reading the Bible.

Even if you know the Bible like the back of your hand, allow the verses you read to challenge your thinking. Imagine ways you can apply what you're reading to your life stage right now. You could read the Bible hundreds of times and still learn something new. That's the power of words inspired by God himself.

While crossword puzzles may just make your brain hurt, God's Word will stimulate you and grow and stretch your mind during this all-important time in your pregnancy. What an amazing brain God gave you!

*Before I formed you in the womb I knew you, before you were born I set you apart. —Jeremiah 1:5a*

# In Your Words

Each person has unique intellectual strengths. What are some of yours?

_____

_____

_____

_____

_____

_____

_____

_____

_____

_____

_____

_____

_____

_____

_____

_____

# WEEK 6
## Life ～ Blood Circulation

*I have come that they may have life,
and have it to the full.*

*JOHN 10:10b*

When a child is born into the world, God draws his
hand out from near his own heart,
and lends something of himself to the parent,
and says, "Keep it till I come."

Henry Ward Beecher

# Mom's Development—Body and Soul

Your hormone levels are rising rapidly. For many women, this means a spike in morning sickness (any-time-of-day sickness for some). Studies show that nausea can indicate a lower risk of miscarriage. But if you're feeling great, don't let that worry you. Many women sail through pregnancy without a stitch of sickness. Consider yourself blessed!

Your baby's blood begins to circulate throughout her body this week. What a miracle! Blood is a symbol of life!

Your own blood will increase in volume throughout your pregnancy. And that life-giving blood will provide your little one with the oxygen and nutrients she needs to thrive in your womb.

Only a creative God could have thought of the concept of blood. And what deep, rich meaning it holds for those who know and follow Christ! Take a moment to thank Jesus for the blood he shed to give you life.

# A Prayer for Baby—Body and Soul

Father, my little baby already has blood circulating through her tiny body. What a symbol of life! I don't often think of the blood running through our veins, but that warm, flowing liquid signifies that my baby is alive!

Oh, Lord, I pray that my child will grow up to be vibrant and full of life. That you will give her such a zeal for living. That she will wake up each morning, energized and excited about what each day holds.

Will you help her feel physically alive, in tune with her body and excited about all it can do? Will you help her feel emotionally alive, in touch with her feelings and all that they entail? Will you help her feel mentally alive, full of questions and ideas about the world around her? And will you help her feel spiritually alive, completely aware of your presence and always growing in her relationship with you?

Thank you for the miracle of blood, Lord. And the gift of life.

In Jesus' name, Amen.

*Before I formed you in the womb I knew you, before you were born I set you apart.* —Jeremiah 1:5a

# Baby's Physical Development

Your baby is now three to five millimeters in length—the size of a peppercorn. Her head is large, and there are dark spots where her eyes and nose are forming. Her fingers and toes are webbed but will soon separate. Her heart is beating, and blood is circulating throughout her body. Her brain is forming three separate parts, and the neural tube is closing.

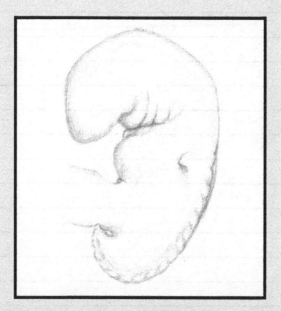

# In Your Words

When do you feel most alive? Write a vivid description.

_____

_____

_____

_____

_____

_____

_____

_____

_____

_____

_____

_____

_____

_____

_____

_____

_____

_____

*Before I formed you in the womb I knew you, before you were born I set you apart. —Jeremiah 1:5a*

# WEEK 7

## Tenderness of Heart

Now that you have purified
yourselves by obeying the truth
so that you have sincere love for your
brothers, love one another deeply,
from the heart.

*1 Peter 1:22*

*Making the decision to have a child is momentous.
It is to decide forever to have your heart go walking
around outside your body.*

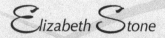

*Elizabeth Stone*

# A Prayer for Baby—Body and Soul

Lord, my baby's heart has been beating for a couple of weeks, but now it can be detected by an ultrasound. I can't wait to see and hear that little heart beating for myself!

My baby's heart has both a right and left chamber now. Every day his inner workings get more and more complex—readying this little person for the outside world.

God, I know that the actual heart isn't where our emotions live—but that's the symbolism we use in our culture. I so want my child to be tender-hearted, never calloused or uncaring. I want him to empathize with the plight of others. I want his heart to be pliable—easily squeezed with joy and even easily constricted with pain. I hate to think of his heart being broken, but a hard heart lacks the capacity to know true love.

Lord, will you give him a soft heart, yet protect it as well? May he have a heart for the things you love.

*In Jesus' name, Amen.*

*Before I formed you in the womb I knew you, before you were born I set you apart. —Jeremiah 1:5a*

# Baby's Physical Development

Your baby is almost half an inch long—the size of a raspberry. His teeth are starting to form, and his brain is developing at a rapid pace. Your little one's heart now has both a left and a right chamber. A transvaginal ultrasound will even be able to detect a heartbeat.

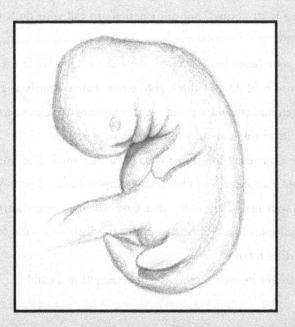

# Mom's Development—Body and Soul

How is this pregnancy treating you so far, Mama? There are a lot of changes going on in your body—even at this early stage.

You might experience an acne breakout—it's high school all over again!—due to a rapid acceleration of hormones. You might get constipated after eating certain foods. And you may get dizzy or light-headed if you stand up too fast.

This is all normal, but don't hesitate to call your doctor with concerns.

Is your heart beating faster these days? Do simple exertions wear you out? As you think about your baby's heartbeat getting stronger, his little heart already separating into two chambers, take a minute to think about your own heart.

Are you ready for your mama's heart to swell? Did you ever imagine your heart could be so tender toward a tiny person you've never even met? Pray today that God will bless your heart with unconditional love and tenderness for this little one—and for any others that follow.

A tender-hearted mother is a priceless gift to a child.

Before I formed you in the womb I knew you, before you were born I set you apart. —Jeremiah 1:5a

# In Your Words

Write a tender love note to your unborn baby.

_____

_____

_____

_____

_____

_____

_____

_____

_____

_____

_____

_____

_____

_____

_____

_____

_____

_____

Tenderness

# WEEK 8

## Attentiveness ∽ Ears

> My sheep listen to my voice;
> I know them,
> and they follow me.
>
> *JOHN 10:27*

*The first duty of love is to listen.*

### Paul Tillich

# Mom's Development—Body and Soul

You're one-fifth of the way through your pregnancy already! You might be feeling bloated and sick to your stomach. This is actually a good thing—for your baby at least. Your digestive process is slowing down, allowing your bloodstream to absorb nutrients more effectively. And your amazing body passes those nutrients on to your growing baby.

So many of your baby's parts are forming now that it's hard to keep track. The presence of your little one's external ears is an exciting development this week.

Think about your own ears for a moment. We don't often stop to consider our ears, do we? Nor do we take time out of our busy schedules to be quiet and just *listen*.

Carve out a few minutes this week to sit still and open your ears. Listen for sounds in nature. Go to a park and listen to the hum of humanity around you. Listen for God's voice of peace in this uncertain time. Let him whisper words of comfort about the weeks and months ahead.

Attentiveness

# A Prayer for Baby—Body and Soul

Lord, my baby's ears are now present on the outside of her little head. What a miracle ears are! I know I take my sense of hearing for granted.

I pray for my child's ears—that they will work correctly and be free from infections and other problems. I pray that she would be attentive to the many sounds around her—the trill of a bird in song, the rush of water in a backyard stream, the steady rain beating against her bedroom window. I pray that she might marvel at the sounds things make—the beautiful rhythm and cadence, melody and harmony of life.

And Lord, may she use her ears for something else, too—to listen to you. You speak to us in that still, small voice, and if we're not ready and listening, we can miss it. Help her not to miss your voice, Lord. Help her to hear your call on her heart and life—and heed it.

*In Jesus' name, I pray for my little one. Amen.*

*Before I formed you in the womb I knew you, before you were born I set you apart. —Jeremiah 1:5a*

# Baby's Physical Development

Your baby is about the size of a kidney bean now—roughly half an inch long. The genitals are developing, but it's still too early to determine Baby's gender. Nerve cells in the brain are beginning to connect. Elbows appear, and bones are starting to harden. The external ears have formed, and Baby is starting to move spontaneously.

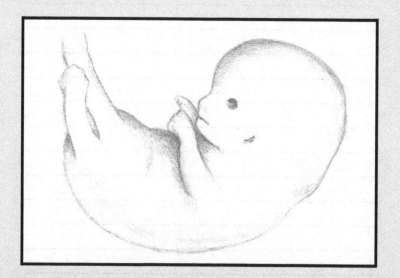

Attentiveness

# In Your Words

For fifteen minutes this week, find a comfortable spot, close your eyes, and just listen. Then briefly record any thoughts or revelations.

_____

_____

_____

_____

_____

_____

_____

_____

_____

_____

_____

_____

_____

_____

_____

_____

_____

_____

*Before I formed you in the womb I knew you, before you were born I set you apart.* —Jeremiah 1:5a

# WEEK 9

## Vision ∾ Eyelids

So we fix our eyes not on what is seen,
but on what is unseen.
For what is seen is temporary,
but what is unseen is eternal.

*2 CORINTHIANS 4:18*

*We see things not as they are but as we are.*

John Milton

# A Prayer for Baby—Body and Soul

God, thank you for painstakingly creating my baby's eyes, and for his eyelids that will protect those eyes as they continue to grow.

Our eyes are so important, Lord, so vital. Eyes allow us to see our world, to become independent, to move and learn and rest. What a travesty it would be to miss out on all the colors and shapes and lights you've created for us. Sight is such a gift. Thank you.

I so want my child to fix his eyes on good and healthy things. Help me to fill his little corner of the world with beauty and brilliance.

And most importantly, help me show him how to fix his eyes on Jesus, to look to you for guidance and wisdom as he travels down life's path. Help me to point out your hand at work in the world at every opportunity.

In Jesus' name, I ask these things. Amen.

Before I formed you in the womb I knew you, before you were born I set you apart. —Jeremiah 1:5a

# Baby's Physical Development

Your tiny one is about the size of a grape now. His basic physical structure is complete, and he's looking more like a human every day. His eyelids are fused shut and will be for the next four months or so. His joints are all in working order now. He can move those little elbows and knees!

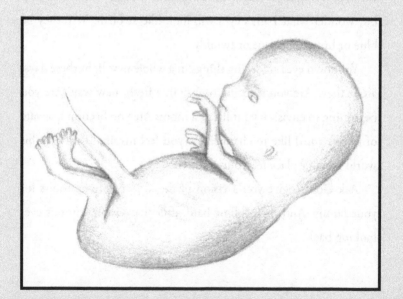

# Mom's Development—Body and Soul

Your pregnancy probably isn't yet visible to the naked eye, but you're definitely starting to feel it—especially when you try to button your jeans!

If your nose has been stuffy, don't worry—you're normal! Nasal congestion and even nosebleeds are common during pregnancy.

Your baby's eyelids are forming and will be fusing shut this week, covering those fragile little eyes until week 27. You can't help but wonder what Baby's eyes will look like at birth. Will they be blue or brown? Serious or twinkly?

Your own eyes are seeing things in a whole new light these days, aren't they? Are you noticing beauty in a fresh, new way? Are you beginning to envision your life as a mom? Are you becoming aware of things you'd like to change? Do you feel inspired to make this world a better place for your children?

Ask God to give you a vision of the kind of life he wants for your family. And then follow hard after that vision without ever looking back.

*Before I formed you in the womb I knew you, before you were born I set you apart.* —Jeremiah 1:5a

# In Your Words

How are you seeing the world differently these days?

_____

_____

_____

_____

_____

_____

_____

_____

_____

_____

_____

_____

_____

_____

_____

_____

_____

_____

*Vision*

# WEEK 10

## Kindness ∽ Upper Lip

Be kind and compassionate to one another,
forgiving each other, just as in Christ
God forgave you.

*EPHESIANS 4:32*

*The kindest word in all the world is the
unkind word, unsaid.*

Author Unknown

# Mom's Development—Body and Soul

You're most likely still pretty tired at this stage of the game. How can a baby so tiny wear you out so much? If you've been battling nausea, you probably still have a few weeks to go, but the end is in sight! Your abdomen may be starting to pooch out a little, depending on your muscle tone and body type. Say good-bye to that waistline!

As your baby's upper lip forms this week (don't you wish you could watch it happen?), take some time to reflect on your own lips. Lips you use for kissing and licking ice cream off of, but most importantly, lips you use to communicate your thoughts and feelings to those around you. It's easy—especially when you're nauseated and exhausted—to be careless about the words that fly off your lips.

Stop and think for a moment before you speak this week. "Will the words I'm about to say be uplifting and kind? Will they be pleasing to the Lord?" If not, don't let them slip past your lips.

*Kindness* 47

# A Prayer for Baby—Body and Soul

Father, my little baby's upper lip will be fully developed this week. I can't imagine how tiny those sweet lips must be.

I pray that my child will use her lips in a way that is pleasing to you, Lord. There is so much potential in such a small part of the body. A person's lips can be a vehicle of negativity and harmful words or they can be used to speak life and hope to others.

May my child speak kindness from her lips from the moment she learns to talk. Will you stop negative words before they even form on those little rosebud lips of hers? Will you cause her to bless others with her choice of words? She will have so much possibility—so many chances to bring joy to so many people. Oh, I want that for her, God.

In Jesus' name, I pray, Amen.

Before I formed you in the womb I knew you, before you were born I set you apart. —Jeremiah 1:5a

# Baby's Physical Development

Your baby is no longer considered an embryo. She's a fetus now. From crown to rump, she's barely an inch long, but the most critical part of her development is already complete. Her tissues and organs are ready to grow and mature in leaps and bounds. Her tail has disappeared, and her external ears and upper lip are completely formed.

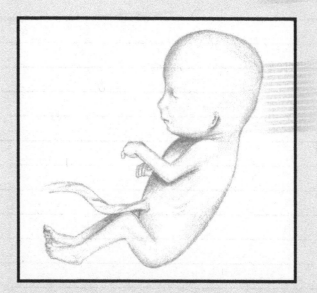

Kindness

# In Your Words

What are some kind words you could speak to specific people this week?

_____

_____

_____

_____

_____

_____

_____

_____

_____

_____

_____

_____

_____

_____

_____

_____

_____

*Before I formed you in the womb I knew you, before you were born I set you apart. —Jeremiah 1:5a*

# WEEK 11

# Confidence ∽ Neck Muscles

Being confident of this, that he who began
a good work in you will carry it on to
completion until the day of Christ Jesus.

*PHILIPPIANS 1:6*

*Nobody can make you feel inferior
without your consent.*

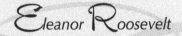

Eleanor Roosevelt

# A Prayer for Baby—Body and Soul

Father, my little one's neck muscles are forming now—so many muscles in his body, and you're lovingly forming each one.

I pray that you will bless him with a strong neck. Even after he's born, I know it will take time before those muscles are strong enough to support the weight of his head. But soon, he'll be holding his head up, moving his head to music, nodding "yes" and shaking his head "no," and bowing his head to pray.

God, I pray that even as a child, he will be able to hold his head high, to be confident in who he is. I don't want him to be cocky or boastful, but to have a healthy pride in the person you created him to be. And may that same neck that holds his head up also help him bow his head low in worship to you, his Creator.

May every single part of his body be used to worship you.

In Jesus' name, Amen.

Before I formed you in the womb I knew you, before you were born I set you apart. —Jeremiah 1:5a

# Baby's Physical Development

Your baby is now fully formed and about the size of a fig. His head is roughly half the size of his body. His skin is still transparent, and some of his bones are starting to harden. The iris of his eyes, his neck muscles, and teensy-tiny fingernails will form this week.

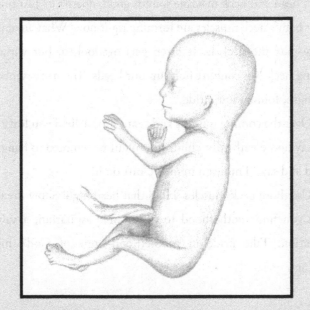

Confidence

# Mom's Development—Body and Soul

Are you afraid you've gained too much or too little weight? Try not to stress. The important thing is to eat healthy foods so your growing baby will get the nutrition he needs.

Headaches are a frequent complaint of pregnant women, due to dramatic changes in hormone levels. Try drinking lots of water and getting plenty of rest.

A head and neck massage sounds good, doesn't it? Just think—your baby's neck muscles are forming right now! What an amazing body part the neck is. It often gets overlooked, but without a strong neck, we couldn't hold up our heads. The neck symbolizes strength, foundation, pride.

Over the coming months and years, especially if you leave a job to stay home with your child, you might be tempted to hang your head and say, "I'm just a mom." Don't do it!

Use those neck muscles. Hold that head high! Show the world that you find motherhood to be a noble aspiration, a valuable ambition. Take pride in motherhood—one of God's highest callings.

Before I formed you in the womb I knew you, before you were born I set you apart. —Jeremiah 1:5a

# In Your Words

Write a brief essay persuading others (and yourself) of the glory and value of motherhood.

_____

_____

_____

_____

_____

_____

_____

_____

_____

_____

_____

_____

_____

_____

_____

_____

_____

_____

# WEEK 12

## Service ∽ Hands

> She opens her arms to the poor and
> extends her hands to the needy.
>
> PROVERBS 31:20

*I am a little pencil in the hand of a writing God who is
sending a love letter to the world.*

Mother Teresa

# Mom's Development—Body and Soul

Are you feeling any relief from your nausea? If not, hopefully soon! Most women find themselves less tired during the second trimester as well.

Your uterus is about the size of a softball now, and your doctor can feel it during an abdominal exam. You might be starting to "show." Your placenta is ready to take over the job of hormone production, and your risk of miscarriage is low.

Your baby's hands are complete, and she's even growing fingernails!

Take a minute to study your own two hands. What do you see? Now, look past your hands' physical appearance, and think about their function. What busy hands we have—so many tasks, so important!

As a mom, your hands will become even more valuable. They'll care for your child, lovingly provide meals for her, hold her face for a kiss, and help meet her every need.

Pray that God will use your hands as loving instruments in the life of your child.

Service

# A Prayer for Baby—Body and Soul

Lord, my baby's hands are completely formed. Your loving hands have carefully crafted hers, and I am in awe.

I'm reminded of the song I sang as a child, "Be careful little hands what you do." Lord, my child's hands have so much potential—to do good and to get in trouble. Will you help her use her hands to love and serve others? Will you give her a heart that loves deeply? Fill her with a strong desire to help those less fortunate than herself?

May she be less worried about keeping her hands physically beautiful and more concerned about attending to the needs of others. She could rake leaves for an elderly neighbor, serve meals at a soup kitchen, care for a younger cousin or sibling.

Bless those little hands, God. May they not be idle, but may they always be reaching out and touching the lives of every person she meets.

In Jesus' name, Amen.

*Before I formed you in the womb I knew you, before you were born I set you apart. —Jeremiah 1:5a*

# Baby's Physical Development

Your baby is about two inches long now, head to bottom. Her face definitely looks more human. Her eyes are moving closer together, and her ears are close to their permanent location on her head. Her hands are complete and growing fingernails. She has acquired more reflexes, and her nerve cells are multiplying rapidly.

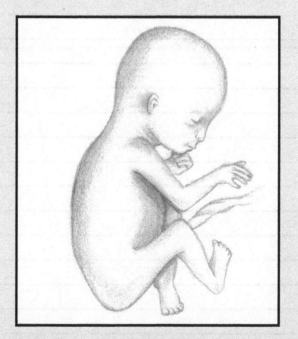

# In Your Words

How can you use your hands this week to bless others?

_____

_____

_____

_____

_____

_____

_____

_____

_____

_____

_____

_____

_____

_____

_____

_____

_____

*Before I formed you in the womb I knew you, before you were born I set you apart. —Jeremiah 1:5a*

# Pleasant Speech ~ Vocal Cords

> *Pleasant words are a honeycomb,*
> *sweet to the soul and healing to the bones.*
>
> PROVERBS 16:24

*If you can't say something nice,*
*don't say anything at all.*

Your Mother

# A Prayer for Baby—Body and Soul

Father, my tiny baby's vocal cords are starting to develop this week. Six months from now, I'll hear that first loud cry—announcing his arrival into the world and assuring us he's healthy and strong.

Oh, God, it won't be long before my little one will be using those vocal cords to say his first word. And then there will be no stopping him! I can't imagine being the mother of a chatty toddler, but I so look forward to that day!

Lord, I know he'll repeat words he hears spoken around him. May my speech be lovely and pure, encouraging and never harsh. May the words of my mouth be pleasing in your sight! And may my little child seek to please you with every word he utters.

Form those precious vocal cords wholly and completely, Lord. He'll need them to sing your praises. Or at least to make a joyful noise unto you all his days. Either way is fine with me!

In Jesus' name I pray, Amen.

Before I formed you in the womb I knew you, before you were born I set you apart. —Jeremiah 1:5a

# Baby's Physical Development

Your baby is about three inches long already—the size of a jumbo shrimp! His head is much more proportional to his body now. He has fingernails and the beginnings of one-of-a-kind fingerprints and footprints. Twenty tiny tooth buds have appeared beneath his gums. He is able to urinate amniotic fluid he has swallowed, and his vocal cords have begun to develop.

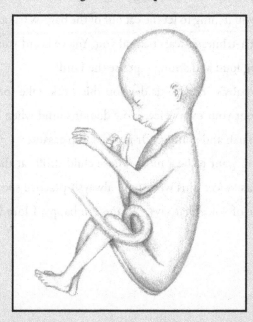

# Mom's Development—Body and Soul

Can you believe you're one-third of the way through your pregnancy? If you're fortunate, your nausea is fading fast. Often called the "honeymoon" of pregnancy, the second trimester is one of renewed energy. Your baby's organs are mostly developed now, and it's time for a welcome break from all your hard work.

Maybe you've kept your pregnancy a secret these long, tiring weeks. Are you itching to let the cat out of the bag? What a relief to put those first-trimester fears behind you. You've heard your baby's heart beating loud and strong—praise the Lord!

As your baby's vocal cords develop this week, take some time to think about your own voice. How does it sound when it leaves your lips? Harsh and grating? Or joyful and pleasant?

Don't you want to be a mom whose child thrills at the sound of his mama's voice? This week (and always!) practice speaking in a sweet tone of voice that says, "I care, I'm happy, I love life, and I love *you*."

Before I formed you in the womb I knew you, before you were born I set you apart. —Jeremiah 1:5a

# In Your Words

What changes do you need to make so that your speech is always pleasant?

_____

_____

_____

_____

_____

_____

_____

_____

_____

_____

_____

_____

_____

_____

_____

_____

_____

_____

Pleasant Speech

# WEEK 14

# Sexual Identity ～ Sex Organ

> But at the beginning of creation God
> "made them male and female."
>
> MARK 10:6

*Where did you come from, baby dear?*
*Out of the everywhere into here.*

## George MacDonald

# Mom's Development—Body and Soul

Your uterus is the size of a grapefruit already. You may have developed a dark line (linea nigra) from your belly button to your pubic bone. Your areola (the dark area of your breast) may have gotten darker and larger as well. You're not the same woman you were three months ago!

Your baby's sex organs are fully differentiated into male or female now. You probably won't find out baby's gender for a few weeks, but if you could peek inside your womb, you'd know!

Speaking of sex, the second trimester is prime lovemaking time. Your nausea should be subsiding; your energy, returning; and you feel curvy but not huge. Make the most of these next few weeks—you won't regret the investment in your marriage!

Sex is an amazing gift God has given you to cultivate with your husband. Purpose in your heart to place a hedge around this gift. Keep your mind and body pure, and remain faithful to your hubby for as long as you both shall live.

# A Prayer for Baby—Body and Soul

Lord, my baby's sexual organs are fully differentiated now. Boy or girl?—one of pregnancy's most exciting questions. You chose our sex before the beginning of time, and our gender defines so much of life for us.

It's an honor to be a woman, and my sexuality has never been as evident as now, when I'm blossoming with child.

I pray that my baby will grow up to be completely content and confident in his or her sexual identity. If I'm carrying a boy, may he embrace his masculinity and seek to become a strong but gentle man who brings honor and glory to his Savior.

If my baby is a girl, may she rejoice in her womanhood and see it not as a burden or a weakness, but as a blessing and a joy.

I will be thrilled with either one, Lord. Help me never to stereotype or put my children in a box, but lovingly encourage them to be exactly who you created them to be.

In Jesus' name, Amen.

68 Before I formed you in the womb I knew you, before you were born I set you apart. —Jeremiah 1:5a

# Baby's Physical Development

Your baby is about three and a half inches long now, crown to rump. By week's end, her arms will be proportional to her body. She is developing fine hair all over her body. She has begun to urinate, she can grasp with her tiny fingers, and she might even be able to suck her thumb! Baby's gender is now apparent, sex orgns are fully differentiated.

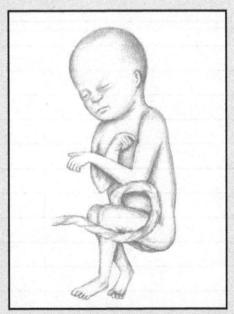

Sexual Identity

# In Your Words

How can you show your husband that your marriage is still a huge priority to you, even while you're pregnant?

_____

_____

_____

_____

_____

_____

_____

_____

_____

_____

_____

_____

_____

_____

_____

_____

_____

*Before I formed you in the womb I knew you, before you were born I set you apart.* —Jeremiah 1:5a

# WEEK 15
# Lifestyle ∽ Digestive Glands

So whether you eat or drink or whatever
you do, do it all for the glory of God.

1 CORINTHIANS 10:31

*By far the most common craving of pregnant
women is not to be pregnant.*

Phyllis Diller

# A Prayer for Baby—Body and Soul

Lord, my little one's digestive glands are completely formed now. Oh, how I pray that every organ and gland continues to work perfectly. I so want my baby to have a healthy body, to eat healthy foods, to use nutrients efficiently, and to smoothly get rid of waste his body doesn't need.

Lord, you have provided us with so many delicious natural foods. I thank you for fresh fruits and vegetables, wholesome grains, and refreshing water to quench our thirst.

I pray that my child will take his health seriously, and that he'll be a good steward of the only body he will ever have.

Help him to see food as something to be enjoyed, but more importantly, as a source of strength and nourishment. Help him to seek out the kinds of food that give him the energy he needs to live up to his fullest potential.

In Jesus' name, Amen.

Before I formed you in the womb I knew you, before you were born I set you apart. —Jeremiah 1:5a

# Baby's Physical Development

Your baby is roughly four inches long now, head to bottom. Sweat glands are starting to appear. His taste buds are forming, and his eyebrows are beginning to grow. His lungs are developing as he inhales and exhales amniotic fluid. His digestive glands are complete, his legs are growing longer than his arms, and he can sense light.

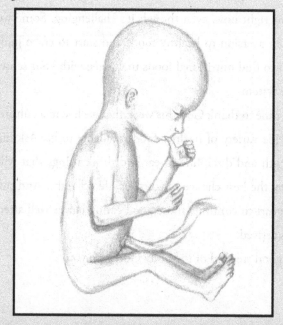

# Mom's Development—Body and Soul

Your uterus is just now peeking over your pubic bone, and your heart is pumping 20 percent more blood than it did before you were pregnant. All of this extra blood will supply your baby with the oxygen he needs to survive.

Your baby's digestive glands are complete, and yours might still be wreaking havoc on your body. Eating nourishing foods is important right now, even though it's challenging. Some women develop an aversion to healthy foods and start to crave junk. Do your best to find nutritional foods that agree with your senses and digestive system.

Take time to thank God this week that we live in a culture with such a wide variety of healthy foods available to us. Ask him for the strength and discipline to eat and drink things that will give your baby the best chance to start his life off right. And purpose in your heart to continue those good eating habits well after your baby has arrived.

Be a good steward of the body God gave you!

*Before I formed you in the womb I knew you, before you were born I set you apart. —Jeremiah 1:5a*

# In Your Words

Describe your idea of a healthy lifestyle. Why do you think such a lifestyle honors God?

_____

_____

_____

_____

_____

_____

_____

_____

_____

_____

_____

_____

_____

_____

_____

_____

_____

_____

# WEEK 16

# Cheerfulness ∽ Facial Muscles

*A cheerful look brings joy to the heart.*

PROVERBS 15:30a

When the first baby laughed for the first time,
the laugh broke into a thousand pieces
and they all went skipping about,
and that was the beginning of fairies.

James Matthew Barrie

# Mom's Development—Body and Soul

It won't be long now before you feel your baby move for the first time. A magical moment indeed! Some women notice this "quickening" as early as this week. Others won't feel anything until 20 weeks or later. Women have compared these first movements to gas bubbles, butterflies, and popcorn popping. As your baby grows, you'll feel definite kicks and punches from within.

Have you noticed your face glowing? The "glow of pregnancy" is no myth. It's caused by increased blood flow to your skin. You may look in the mirror and smile at your reflection, feeling more beautiful than ever.

Someone else is smiling this week—your baby! Her facial muscles are developing, and she's busy trying them out—smiling, squinting, frowning.

Take a moment to think about how often you smile. Is your countenance characteristically happy? Does your zest for life show on your face? Can people see the joy of the Lord etched in your features?

"Rejoice in the Lord always!" the Bible says. Let's see those dimples and pearly whites!

# A Prayer for Baby—Body and Soul

Father, my baby is developing facial muscles this week. Is she registering emotion? Smiling and frowning for a reason? What an amazing thought!

I would give anything to watch her little face right now. To see it scrunch up in a frown, erupt in a grin, squint in the sunlight.

God, I want her to be a happy baby, a happy child, a happy teenager. I pray that she will be known for her smile, not her scowl. That she will be a joy to know, that her happiness will be contagious. That her smile will bless everyone she meets.

I pray that her face is a reflection of the joy she has found in you. That people will want to know why she's so happy and that she will be ready and willing to share the reason. Help her to tell them she was created with a purpose, is loved by the God of the universe, and has a personal relationship with his Son, Jesus Christ.

*In that Son's name, I pray. Amen.*

*Before I formed you in the womb I knew you, before you were born I set you apart. —Jeremiah 1:5a*

# Baby's Physical Development

Your baby is four and a half inches long now and weighs roughly three ounces. In the next three weeks, she'll experience a huge growth spurt. Her weight will double, and she'll grow a few inches. Her circulatory system and urinary tract are working. She is using her facial muscles—squinting, smiling, and frowning.

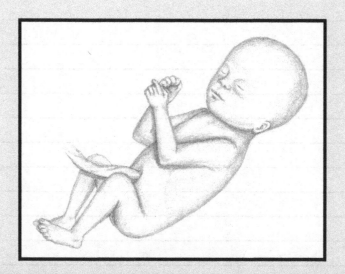

# In Your Words

Make a list of things that bring a smile to your face.

_____

_____

_____

_____

_____

_____

_____

_____

_____

_____

_____

_____

_____

_____

_____

_____

_____

*Before I formed you in the womb I knew you, before you were born I set you apart. —Jeremiah 1:5a*

# WEEK 17

## Individuality ∽ Fingerprints

*I praise you because I am fearfully and wonderfully made; your works are wonderful, I know that full well.*

PSALM 139:14

*I am only one, but I am one.*
*I cannot do everything, but I can do something.*
*And I will not let what I cannot do*
*interfere with what I can do.*

## Edward Everett Hale

# A Prayer for Baby—Body and Soul

Finishing up Baby's fingerprints and toe prints is on your creation agenda this week, Lord. I wonder how in the world you engrave those swirls and whorls and lines on those tiny little fingers and toes. A masterpiece that you will never again replicate exactly. I stand in awe.

Oh, God, would you help my child embrace his uniqueness? I know that peer pressure starts at an early age. I know he's going to be faced with the desire to "be like everybody else." Will you help me instill in him an appreciation for his distinctive traits, that combination of qualities that sets him apart?

Help him to delight in who he is, delight in who others are, and be thankful that you bestowed different gifts upon us all. There are few greater blessings in life than to be perfectly content with who we are and what you have given us.

I can't wait to meet this little baby that you've fearfully and wonderfully made!

*In Jesus' name, I pray for my child. Amen.*

*Before I formed you in the womb I knew you, before you were born I set you apart.* —Jeremiah 1:5a

# Baby's Physical Development

Your baby is big enough to kick you now—you may or may not be able to feel it. He is developing pads on his fingertips and toes. The umbilical cord is getting longer and thicker as your baby grows and needs more food. The placenta and baby are almost the same size.

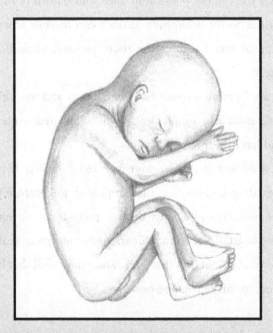

*Individuality*

# Mom's Development—Body and Soul

Increased secretions are the name of the game during the second trimester. There's just no polite way to say it. You might be sweating more, experiencing nasal congestion, and stocking up on pantiliners. This is all perfectly normal and is caused by the increase in your body's blood volume. Inconvenient, yes, but there isn't much you can do. It will stop once your baby is born.

Continue to eat healthfully, make room in your schedule for some type of exercise, and take those prenatal vitamins. You're doing great!

Pads are forming on your baby's fingertips and toes this week. Soon their exact and unique design will be apparent—no baby in the world has fingerprints like yours.

Take a minute to ponder your own individuality. There is no one on earth quite like you. The temptation to compare yourself to other women—especially during pregnancy—is very real. Don't give in to it! Focus on your strengths, not your weaknesses. Embrace your uniqueness this week, and praise God that he loved you enough to make you one-of-a-kind.

Before I formed you in the womb I knew you, before you were born I set you apart. —Jeremiah 1:5a

# In Your Words

What makes you a unique individual? Make a list of traits and then thank God for each one.

_____

_____

_____

_____

_____

_____

_____

_____

_____

_____

_____

_____

_____

_____

_____

_____

_____

*Individuality*

# WEEK 18

## Walk ∽ Legs

He has showed you, O man, what is good.
And what does the LORD require of
you? To act justly and to love mercy
and to walk humbly with your God.

MICAH 6:8

*Every action in our lives touches on some chord*
*that will vibrate in eternity.*

Edwin Hubbel Chapin

# Mom's Development—Body and Soul

Are you wearing maternity clothes yet? As cute as they are, you don't want to buy too many at this point. You'll probably be going up a size or two in the next few months.

You might be having trouble sleeping. It's not always easy to find a comfortable position. Many pregnant women use body pillows or a pillow between their legs. Always sleep on your side, preferably your left side. When you lie on your back or right side, your uterus can compress one of the major veins that carries blood to your heart.

Your baby's legs are lengthening this week. How are your own legs holding up? You might experience leg cramps, swelling, or just general tiredness from carrying around all that extra weight.

Take some time this week to go for a walk. And while you're walking, think about the path you're taking in life. Are you following after God? Are you letting him lead you? Do you trust him to lead you down the path that is best for you?

If you've wandered, get back on the trail!

# A Prayer for Baby—Body and Soul

My baby's legs are lengthening this week, Lord. Her bones are getting harder and longer. I marvel at how you cause things to grow.

As I think of baby legs, I think of little ones learning to stand and then taking a step and then walking. And once they can walk, there's no stopping them.

God, I want my child's legs to be physically fit and strong. But more important, I want her to use her legs to follow you. I want her to physically walk with you all of her days—in her actions, the places she goes, the things she does. But also spiritually—making choices that honor you, seeking to please you always.

I know it isn't always easy walking down that "narrow road." The pressure to conform will be high. Will you help me build up spiritual muscle in my child, so that walking with you is something she desires and is able to do?

In Jesus' name, Amen.

Before I formed you in the womb I knew you, before you were born I set you apart. —Jeremiah 1:5a

# Baby's Physical Development

Your baby is about five and a half inches this week, crown to rump. You can see her blood vessels through her skin, and her ears are sticking out from her head. Her body is forming myelin (a protective coating) around her nerves, and this will continue until her first birthday. Her legs are lengthening, and her body length is catching up with her head size.

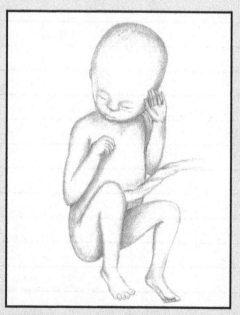

WEEK 18 • WALK

# In Your Words

"Walking with the Lord" can seem like such an abstract concept sometimes. What does it mean to you?

_____

_____

_____

_____

_____

_____

_____

_____

_____

_____

_____

_____

_____

_____

_____

_____

_____

_____

90 *Before I formed you in the womb I knew you, before you were born I set you apart.* —Jeremiah 1:5a

# WEEK 19
# Foundation ～ Feet

> Make level paths for your feet and take
> only ways that are firm.
>
> PROVERBS 4:26

*The greatest gift a parent can give a child is
unconditional love. As a child wanders and strays,
finding his bearings, he needs a sense of absolute love
from a parent. There's nothing wrong with tough love,
as long as the love is unconditional.*

George Herbert Walker Bush

# A Prayer for Baby—Body and Soul

Lord, this might be the week I feel my baby kick me. His feet are getting stronger, and he's learning how to use them. What a miracle.

I pray that you will bless my child's feet, Father. I pray that you will grant him firm footing as he walks through life. It says in the book of Psalms that those who love your Word will have great peace, and nothing will make them stumble. I pray that you would instill in my child a love for your Word and keep him from stumbling all of his days.

Will you help me establish a firm foundation for him—a home and family that are solid and sure? Will you help him make good choices and avoid disastrous mistakes? Will you keep him off the slippery slope and lead him on firm, level paths?

Those tiny feet will grow bigger and bigger with each passing year. Please keep them moving in the right direction.

In Jesus' name, Amen.

Before I formed you in the womb I knew you, before you were born I set you apart. —Jeremiah 1:5a

# Baby's Physical Development

Your baby is getting bigger, and you can probably feel those tiny feet kicking by now. Your baby is covered in a white coating called vernix that protects his delicate skin. His permanent teeth buds are starting to form behind the milk teeth buds. Brown fat is also starting to develop. This keeps your baby warm after he's born.

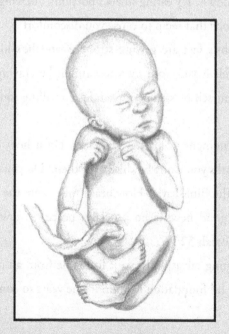

# Mom's Development—Body and Soul

Your blood pressure might be lower than usual during your second trimester. Your cardiovascular system is changing dramatically. If you stand up too fast, you might get dizzy.

Heartburn is also common. Your uterus is pushing against your stomach, and the movement of food through your digestive system has slowed down. Try eating smaller portions, chewing antacids, or avoiding foods that seem to cause you discomfort.

Your baby's feet are getting stronger, and he's kicking more. Have you felt it yet? Your own feet might be craving a massage. Consider yourself blessed if you can find a willing soul to give you one!

Take a moment to look at your feet. Do it now, because in a couple months you won't be able to see them! Do you think they're beautiful? The Bible says, "How beautiful . . . are the feet of those who bring good news, who proclaim peace, . . . who proclaim salvation" (Isaiah 52:7).

Proclaiming salvation to your little one from an early age will provide a solid foundation for him in the years to come.

Before I formed you in the womb I knew you, before you were born I set you apart. —Jeremiah 1:5a

# In Your Words

What are some of the ways you hope to provide a firm foundation for your child?

_____

_____

_____

_____

_____

_____

_____

_____

_____

_____

_____

_____

_____

_____

_____

_____

_____

_____

# WEEK 20
# Womanhood ∼ Gender

> A wife of noble character who can find?
> She is worth far more than rubies.
> Her husband has full confidence in her
> and lacks nothing of value. . . .
> Her children arise and call her blessed;
> her husband also, and he praises her.
>
> *PROVERBS 31:10–11, 28*

*What are little girls made of?*
*What are little girls made of?*
*Sugar and spice, and all that's nice,*
*That's what little girls are made of.*

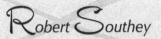
Robert Southey

# Mom's Development—Body and Soul

You are officially halfway through your pregnancy! Can you believe it? Maybe you've already scheduled an ultrasound. If you want to know your baby's gender, you should be able to find out with little difficulty.

The top of your uterus is at belly button level. Strangers can tell that you're pregnant now. They might even give you a knowing smile and extend extra courtesy to you in your "condition." You're enjoying the attention, aren't you?

Pregnancy is definitely a time to celebrate being a woman. If you're carrying a baby girl, her uterus is already formed, she's beginning to develop a vagina, and she has six million eggs in her ovaries. She's a little woman!

Take some time this week to reflect on your womanhood. What does it mean to be a woman? What are some strengths you have because of your gender?

Just think: When God created you, he wanted you to be a woman. He made you a woman on purpose and has great plans for your life as his daughter. Praise him!

# A Prayer for Baby—Body and Soul

Lord, I'll be so thrilled with either a girl or a boy. I know my baby's gender will largely determine the course of my life as a mom. I'm ready for anything.

Lord, if my baby is a girl, you've already given her all the body parts she needs to grow into a woman. Of course, she'll have to mature and go through puberty, but everything she needs is in place. What a miracle.

Oh, I pray that my baby will embrace her God-given sexuality. Give her a fierce desire to keep her mind and body pure. I pray for her future mate, that she'll save her virginity for him on their wedding night. Will you bless her precious womb with children? After carrying a child for just 20 weeks, I want any woman who so desires to experience this miracle for themselves—especially my own daughter.

Lord, help her to love being a woman—and give her the strength to be exactly the woman you want her to be.

*In Jesus' name, Amen.*

*Before I formed you in the womb I knew you, before you were born I set you apart. —Jeremiah 1:5a*

# Baby's Physical Development

For the second twenty weeks, Baby's measurements will be taken from head to toe, instead of head to bottom. In that case, your banana-sized baby is about ten inches long. If you're carrying a girl, her vagina is beginning to develop. Her uterus and ovaries are already formed.

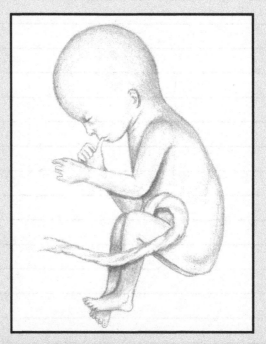

# In Your Words

What do you love most about being a woman?

_____

_____

_____

_____

_____

_____

_____

_____

_____

_____

_____

_____

_____

_____

_____

_____

_____

*Before I formed you in the womb I knew you, before you were born I set you apart. —Jeremiah 1:5a*

# WEEK 21

## Protection ∽ Fat

> You are my hiding place; you will protect
> me from trouble and surround me
> with songs of deliverance.
>
> *PSALM 32:7*

*Who fed me from her gentle breast*
*And hushed me in her arms to rest,*
*And on my cheek sweet kisses prest?*
*My Mother.*

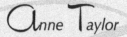

Anne Taylor

# A Prayer for Baby—Body and Soul

My little baby is adding fat to his bones this week, Lord. How exciting! This fat will keep him warm when he leaves my cozy womb and enters this big, cold world. These layers of fat will cushion and protect him—and give me something to kiss and pinch.

Lord, I pray that you will always keep my child warm and protected. I thank you that he will be born in a warm place and live in a warm home. I thank you that we can afford diapers, clean clothing, and blankets. And he'll have his mama and so many other loved ones to snuggle with around the clock.

God, will you send your angels to protect my darling child? As much as I'd love to be there for him every second of his life, I know I can't be. Even if I could, some things are beyond my control. Help me to trust you to protect my little one. He already means the world to me.

In Jesus' name, I pray. Amen.

Before I formed you in the womb I knew you, before you were born I set you apart. —Jeremiah 1:5a

# Baby's Physical Development

Your baby weighs a whopping twelve ounces now. He has fully developed eyebrows and eyelids. You've most likely felt him move at this point—at all times of the day and night. He is getting meat on his bones, fat that will help keep him warm outside the womb.

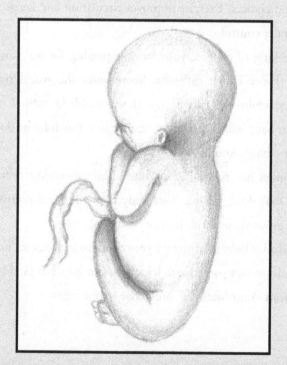

Protection

# Mom's Development—Body and Soul

You've officially begun the second half of your pregnancy. What a milestone! Be sure you're getting exercise, but don't do anything too crazy. Your ligaments are more relaxed, and you're more susceptible to injury. Walking, swimming, and prenatal aerobics are good choices. Exercise improves circulation and keeps weight gain under control.

Speaking of weight, your baby is putting fat on those little bones. Every baby's different. Some enter the world tiny and scrawny, while others are born with squeezable fat rolls.

Your baby will be perfect no matter how much fat he does—or doesn't—have. And so are you.

Women are notorious for unhealthily obsessing over being thin. Don't do it, Mama. Your body is cradling and nourishing a living, growing, precious human being right now.

And after Baby is born, take your time getting back to "normal." Our culture says you have to look a certain way, but God looks at your heart. Your beautiful, protective mama heart.

Before I formed you in the womb I knew you, before you were born I set you apart. —Jeremiah 1:5a

# In Your Words

Make a list of all the reasons your womb is such a safe, protected place.

_____

_____

_____

_____

_____

_____

_____

_____

_____

_____

_____

_____

_____

_____

_____

_____

_____

_____

_____

_____

_____

Protection

# WEEK 22

## Listening ∽ Hearing

> *Everyone should be quick to listen,*
> *slow to speak and slow to become angry.*
>
> JAMES 1:19b

*Courage is what it takes to stand up and speak;*
*courage is also what it takes to sit down and listen.*

## Winston Churchill

# Mom's Development—Body and Soul

Have you had any Braxton Hicks contractions yet? These abdomen-squeezing contractions are usually painless, and they won't harm your baby. If you feel pain, or if the contractions increase in intensity and frequency, let your doctor know.

Unless Doc says otherwise, feel free to enjoy sex with your hubby as long as you can. If you've been amorous of late, it's probably due to the increased flow of blood to your genitals.

Your baby can now hear sounds from outside the womb. Isn't that amazing? You can talk to her now, and when she's born, she'll recognize your voice!

Before long she'll be talking back! Purpose in your heart to be the kind of mom who truly listens to her child. When she asks a million questions, listen. When she stretches accounts of her day into twenty-minute monologues, listen. When she has a problem, listen. When she's sharing her hopes and dreams, listen.

Your heavenly Father is always there to listen to you. Always be there, with bended ear, for your child.

Listening

# A Prayer for Baby—Body and Soul

Lord, my baby can hear sounds outside of my womb now! She can hear my voice. I can start communicating with my little one weeks before she enters the world. What a privilege!

Father, as she grows, will you keep those ears of hers open? Will you help her to hear the cries of the poor, the forsaken, the helpless? Will you give her a sensitivity to others and a heart that wants to help?

So often, I turn a deaf ear to the needs of those around me and focus on my own selfish desires. I don't want to be like that anymore! And I don't want my child to be like that either.

Help me to show her what it means to be in tune with others, to care about them more than you care about yourself. From an early age, may she be aware of those who need a tender touch— and then reach out to touch them.

*In Jesus' name, I pray. Amen.*

*Before I formed you in the womb I knew you, before you were born I set you apart. —Jeremiah 1:5a*

# Baby's Physical Development

Your baby weighs nearly a pound now. The brain and nerve endings have developed enough for your little one to feel touch. Her taste buds have started to form on her tongue, and she can hear sounds from the outside world. In a few short weeks, your baby will be able to survive outside the womb.

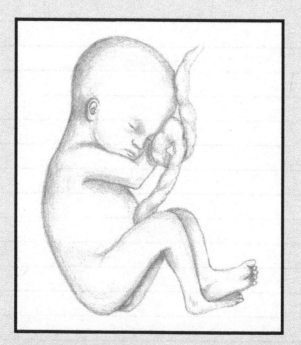

*Listening*

# In Your Words

Who do you know who could use a listening ear? Write down a plan of action for listening wholeheartedly to that person for a chunk of time this week.

_____

_____

_____

_____

_____

_____

_____

_____

_____

_____

_____

_____

_____

_____

_____

_____

_____

_____

*Before I formed you in the womb I knew you, before you were born I set you apart.* —Jeremiah 1:5a

# WEEK 23

## Rest ∽ Sleep

Come to me, all you who are weary and
burdened, and I will give you rest.
Take my yoke upon you and learn from me,
for I am gentle and humble in heart,
and you will find rest for your souls.
For my yoke is easy, and my burden is light.

*MATTHEW 11:28–30*

*Drop Thy still dews of quietness,*
*Till all our strivings cease;*
*Take from our souls the strain and stress,*
*And let our ordered lives confess*
*The beauty of Thy peace.*

John Greenleaf Whittier

# A Prayer for Baby—Body and Soul

Father, my baby's eyelids are completely formed. These fragile and delicate pieces of skin will enable him to get the sleep a growing baby needs.

As he grows, rest will continue to be an important part of his life. I know little ones are so active and have all kinds of energy, but they need rest too! Help me to gently remind him when he needs some downtime and to enforce it even when he's unwilling.

Help us to make the Sabbath an important part of our week as a family. You've wired us in such a way that we need regular rest. Help us to resist the temptation to go, go, go twenty-four hours a day, seven days a week.

Show my child that you'll take care of him while he rests and that you won't let him fall behind in school, sports, and life when he takes time to rest each week in you.

*In Jesus' name, I pray for my precious child. Amen.*

*Before I formed you in the womb I knew you, before you were born I set you apart. —Jeremiah 1:5a*

# Baby's Physical Development

Your baby weighs just a little over a pound. His eyelids are completely formed, as are all ten of his fingernails. His pancreas has started producing insulin. The lungs are beginning to develop surfactant, a substance that will help baby's lungs expand after birth. His patterns of sleep and activity are becoming more regular.

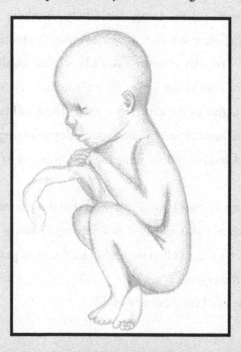

# Mom's Development—Body and Soul

Your prenatal visits are getting more exciting now, aren't they? Finding out how much you've gained, hearing your baby's heartbeat, getting measured to see if you're right on track. Don't worry if you measure a little "too big" or "too small." Every woman is different.

Make sure you're eating healthfully, drinking plenty of water, getting some exercise, and enjoying each moment of your pregnancy. Write things down—you'll be so glad you did!

Your baby's eyelids are now completely formed. Those thin little flaps of skin give us the capacity to sleep. There will be countless times in your future when you sing your little one to sleep, caressing his forehead and his eyelids, watching him in awe as he slips off to dreamland.

Take time to thank God this week for the gift of rest. And take time to rest yourself! Rest is a blessing he wants us to take advantage of—and so often we neglect it. You need periods of rest now more than ever.

Bless the Lord for creating eyelids!

*Before I formed you in the womb I knew you, before you were born I set you apart. —Jeremiah 1:5a*

# In Your Words

You may think you don't have time to rest right now, but you need to make the time. Where and how can you carve out time to rest this week?

_____

_____

_____

_____

_____

_____

_____

_____

_____

_____

_____

_____

_____

_____

_____

_____

# Truth ∽ Swallow

Jesus said, "If you hold to my teaching,
you are really my disciples.
Then you will know the truth,
and the truth will set you free."

*JOHN 8:31b–32*

*If you tell the truth you don't have to
remember anything.*

Mark Twain

# Mom's Development—Body and Soul

Your uterus is about the size of a soccer ball. No hiding it now! As your abdomen and breasts swell and stretch, your skin will itch. Lotions may help.

You might be given a glucose screening test between 24 and 28 weeks. This test checks for gestational diabetes, a high-blood-sugar condition common during pregnancy. No needles or blood involved, just a sugary drink.

As you swallow that bottle of sugar, your baby can swallow inside your womb! What an important body function!

Swallowing can be taken figuratively as well—as in swallowing harmful or false words before you say them. This will be important for you as a mom. As your child gets older and does things that anger you, you'll need to weigh your words before spitting them out. A mom's words can build up a child or they can wound her deeply. And lies should have no place at all in your speech—or in your heart.

Ask God this week to help you speak only words of love and truth. Ask yourself three questions before you open your mouth. Is it true? Is it kind? Is it necessary?

# A Prayer for Baby—Body and Soul

Lord, my baby can swallow now! A reflex I take for granted so often. Will you be with my baby right now as she develops all the functions she needs to survive outside of me?

God, I know my child will face countless opportunities as she grows older to lie instead of tell the truth. Will you give her the courage to swallow lies before they leave her lips? To speak only words that are true and right? Will you keep her from half-truths and bending the truth? Show her that lying makes things worse in the long run. It is always best to tell the truth—even when there are consequences.

Help me to teach her your truth. She'll eventually have to figure things out on her own, but I can give her a firm foundation by introducing her to your word at an early age. "Keep falsehood and lies far from me," King Solomon prays in the book of Proverbs. I pray the same thing for my child, Father.

In Jesus' name, Amen.

Before I formed you in the womb I knew you, before you were born I set you apart. —Jeremiah 1:5a

# Baby's Physical Development

Your baby is almost a foot long now and weighs about one and a quarter pounds. That's not much weight for twelve inches of baby, but she's filling out more every day. Her taste buds are developing, her brain is growing, she's putting on fat, and she can swallow. What an amazing baby!

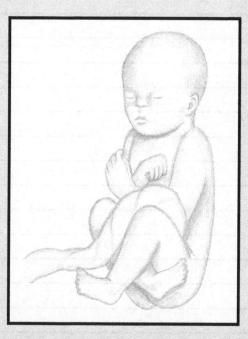

Truth

## In Your Words

Are you often tempted to speak in anger or fudge the truth? Write a prayer asking God to help you improve in these areas.

_____

_____

_____

_____

_____

_____

_____

_____

_____

_____

_____

_____

_____

_____

_____

_____

_____

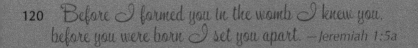

120  Before I formed you in the womb I knew you, before you were born I set you apart. —Jeremiah 1:5a

# Gift of Food ~ Taste Buds

> Taste and see that the LORD is good.
>
> *PSALM 34:8a*

*A newborn is merely a small, noisy object, slightly fuzzy at one end, with no distinguishing marks to speak of except a mouth. But to its immediate family it is without question the most phenomenal, the most astonishing, the most absolutely unparalleled thing that has yet occurred in the entire history of the planet.*

Irving Cobb

# A Prayer for Baby—Body and Soul

God, my baby's taste buds are completely developed now. He can use his little tongue to taste things! I am amazed at how taste buds work in connection with the brain, registering likes and dislikes.

At first, there won't be much variety in my baby's diet, but then I'll have the privilege of introducing him to his first fruits, vegetables, and grains. I know I'll have some measure of control over what he eats, but his taste buds are unique to him. He'll like what he likes.

God, would you help me to expose my child to a wide variety of healthy foods? Would you bless him with taste buds that embrace foods of all kinds, from all cultures? I want him to be well rounded, to be willing to try anything once, and to be comfortable eating the food in any part of the world.

Help me to teach him that every good and perfect gift comes from you—even food—and model a spirit of gratitude for each gift.

*In Jesus' name, Amen.*

*Before I formed you in the womb I knew you, before you were born I set you apart. —Jeremiah 1:5a*

# Baby's Physical Development

Your baby weighs about one and a half pounds now and is thirteen and a half inches long. You're noticing stronger movement every day, and you can probably tell when your baby is napping as well. He can hear with his ears and taste with his tongue, and he's growing hair. Every day, his little body becomes more proportional.

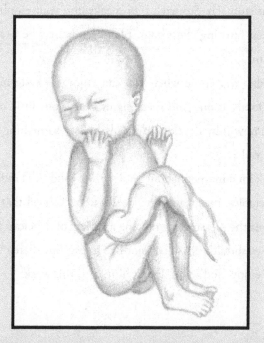

# Mom's Development—Body and Soul

Pregnancy definitely has both its perks and its downsides. One good thing is that your hair has more body. You're not growing more hair; it just isn't falling out as quickly.

And some bad news? Heartburn. The progesterone in your body slows the emptying of your stomach and relaxes the valve into your stomach. Stomach acid sneaks into your esophagus and causes that burning chest pain. Bland foods may be best for you at this time.

The day will come when you can enjoy the taste of all your favorite foods again. And speaking of taste, your little one's taste buds are now fully developed! If only he had something delicious to snack on!

Think for a moment about God's gift of food. All kinds of fruits and vegetables, meats and grains. We are so blessed that God has allowed us the pleasure of enjoying a variety of delicious foods. Of course, we should eat to live, not live to eat, but there's no reason we can't enjoy God's gift. Thank him for it this week.

Before I formed you in the womb I knew you, before you were born I set you apart. —Jeremiah 1:5a

# In Your Words

Besides food, what other common, everyday gifts has God given you?

_____

_____

_____

_____

_____

_____

_____

_____

_____

_____

_____

_____

_____

_____

_____

_____

_____

# WEEK 26

## Image of God ∽ Face

> Then God said, "Let us make man
> in our image, in our likeness."
>
> *GENESIS 1:26*

*I've never seen a smiling face that was not beautiful.*

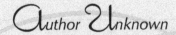

*Author Unknown*

# Mom's Development—Body and Soul

Between the weight gain and those pregnancy hormones, your body can feel a bit out of whack. Your joints and ligaments have loosened. Your center of gravity has shifted. Everything seems to take more effort than it used to. Do your best to maintain good posture. Keep up the mild exercise. And stretch your muscles a couple of times a day.

Make sure you're familiar with the warning signs of preeclampsia—a dangerous condition that occurs in 5 percent of pregnancies. Watch for sudden weight gain, blurry vision, sudden headaches, upper abdominal pain, and swelling in your hands and feet.

Of course, some swelling is normal, especially in your face. Some women go through pregnancy showing only "out front." Others look pregnant from the forehead down.

Your pregnant face is beautiful, no matter how "full." Let it reflect the glow in your heart—the joy you feel because of impending motherhood. The joy you feel as a daughter of the King. You were made in the image of your heavenly Father. May those around you see his love in your features.

Image of God

# A Prayer for Baby—Body and Soul

Lord, according to the "experts," my baby's face has assumed the appearance of a full-term infant at birth. The face she has now is the face she'll be born with! I'm so thankful for the technology of 4-D ultrasounds, but I so want to meet her in person, face-to-face!

I know my child will be beautiful to her mommy. But more importantly, she'll be beautiful to you, because you created her in your own image. I don't pretend to know all that that means, but what an amazing thing. We were created in your image.

She might look like her mom or her dad, but the key to a fulfilling life is to resemble *you*. Help her to follow after you all of her days, to want to imitate you, to grow more and more like you.

Help her to live her life like one made in God's image. And continue to show her every day what that will look like.

*In Jesus' name, Amen.*

*Before I formed you in the womb I knew you, before you were born I set you apart. —Jeremiah 1:5a*

# Baby's Physical Development

Your baby is fourteen inches long. She is starting to make breathing movements, continuing to develop her lungs. She can respond to touch, and her face now looks like the face of a full-term newborn. Tiny nerve pathways in her ears are developing, refining her sense of hearing.

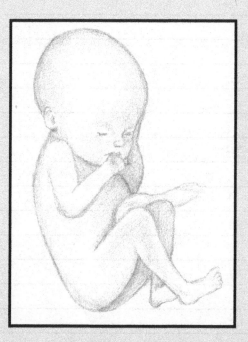

Image of God 129

# In Your Words

What do you think it means to be created in God's image? How might this play out in your everyday life?

_____

_____

_____

_____

_____

_____

_____

_____

_____

_____

_____

_____

_____

_____

_____

_____

_____

_____

Before I formed you in the womb I knew you, before you were born I set you apart. —Jeremiah 1:5a

# *Appreciation* ∽ **B**reath

> *Let everything that has breath*
> *praise the* LORD.
>
> PSALM 150:6a

*We can do no great things,*
*only small things with great love.*

Mother Teresa

# A Prayer for Baby—Body and Soul

Lord, my little one is taking some practice breaths inside of me. Isn't that unreal? I must confess, I rarely take time to stop and pay attention to the breaths I take. I wonder how many times I breathe in and out in one minute, one hour, one day. Without you, I couldn't take a single one.

It says in the Psalms, "Let everything that has breath praise the Lord." There are so many ways we can praise you, for as long as we have breath. Father, I pray that my child will be aware of you at all times. I pray that he'll appreciate you and the many gifts you've lavished on us. May he demonstrate his appreciation in tangible ways each day.

"Don't waste your breath" is a worn-out cliché, but I do pray that my child never wastes his breath. I pray that he considers carefully what he wants to spend his time and efforts doing. And I pray he chooses to honor you by living a life of gratitude.

In Jesus' name, Amen.

Before I formed you in the womb I knew you, before you were born I set you apart. —Jeremiah 1:5a

# Baby's Physical Development

Your baby weighs about two pounds now and is taking his first breaths in utero. Countless babies have been born at two pounds and survived—even thrived. Your baby's heartbeat is getting louder and stronger, and he's very active. His wrinkled, raisinlike skin (he lives in a bathtub!) will stay that way until a couple of weeks after he's born.

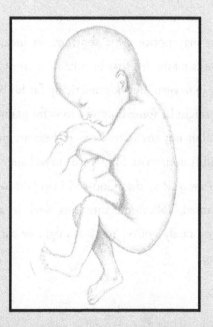

Appreciation

# Mom's Development—Body and Soul

Congratulations! You made it! To the third trimester, that is. Your baby is stronger and more active. You'll start to put on more weight each week—and this is okay! Changing hormones and your baby pushing on your bladder might cause a little bit of urine to leak out at inconvenient times, such as when coughing, laughing, or running. Ask your practitioner what you can do to minimize this problem.

While you may notice some shortness of breath these days, your little one is taking his first breaths in utero. Of course, he's not breathing in oxygen, but he's practicing for his big day!

Breathing might be something you took for granted before you got pregnant, but not anymore. In fact, there are probably many things you didn't appreciate fully until they changed, got harder, or were taken away. Pray that God will help you to take nothing in life for granted. Take some time this week to appreciate the little things you rarely notice. You just might be surprised at how blessed you are.

Before I formed you in the womb I knew you, before you were born I set you apart. —Jeremiah 1:5a

# In Your Words

What are some little things in life you want to appreciate this week?

_____

_____

_____

_____

_____

_____

_____

_____

_____

_____

_____

_____

_____

_____

_____

_____

_____

*Appreciation*

# Future ∽ Dreams

> "For I know the plans I have for you,"
> declares the LORD,
> "plans to prosper you and not to harm you,
> plans to give you hope and a future."
>
> *JEREMIAH 29:11*

If a child is to keep alive his inborn sense of wonder,
he needs the companionship of at least one adult
who can share it, rediscovering with him the joy,
excitement, and mystery of the world we live in.

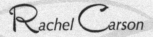

Rachel Carson

# Mom's Development—Body and Soul

So much on your mind right now. The third trimester is when you start feeling the crunch, when you realize, "My baby will be here before I know it. Am I ready?"

You need a name for your baby (two, if you don't know the gender). You probably have a nursery you want decorated. If you intend to have a labor plan, now is a good time to write it down.

You might be spending a lot of time dreaming these days—both during the day and while you sleep. Guess what! Your baby is starting to dream too! If only you could take a peek at those dreams. How can she dream about a world she's never seen?

What kind of dreams do you have for your future? For your child's future? Do you sense a peace about those dreams? Do they seem to line up with what God dreams for you? Pray this week that God will help you recognize his dreams for your future—and then pursue them with all of your heart.

*Future*

# A Prayer for Baby—Body and Soul

Lord, my baby is starting to dream already! Don't ask me how doctors and scientists know these kinds of things. I'll just have to trust them. But I must admit it boggles my mind that a baby can dream before she even leaves the womb.

I pray that my child will dream big dreams for her future. I pray that you will bless her with a healthy confidence in who she is. I pray that she won't be afraid to pursue anything her heart desires out of life. And I hope and pray that her dreams will align with the ones you've had for her since before time began.

Lord, bless her as she sleeps with peaceful dreams. And when she's awake, help her to form an exciting and positive vision for her future. Do big things through her, God. I can't wait to see what you have planned!

In Jesus' name, Amen.

Before I formed you in the womb I knew you, before you were born I set you apart. —Jeremiah 1:5a

# Baby's Physical Development

Remember how your baby's eyelids have been fused shut for all these many weeks? Well, they're beginning to open and close! She even has a new set of eyelashes! Her brain tissue continues to develop, she begins to dream, and she's starting to stick to a distinctive pattern of movement and sleep. She weighs in at over two pounds and is nearly fifteen inches long.

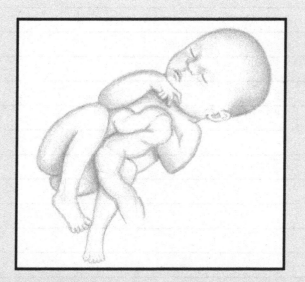

# In Your Words

What big dreams do you have for your child? For yourself?

_____

_____

_____

_____

_____

_____

_____

_____

_____

_____

_____

_____

_____

_____

_____

_____

_____

*Before I formed you in the womb I knew you, before you were born I set you apart. —Jeremiah 1:5a*

# WEEK 29
# *Intimacy ❧ Bone Marrow*

For you created my inmost being; you knit

me together in my mother's womb.

*PSALM 139:13*

*All that I have seen teaches me to trust God*
*for all I have not seen.*

*Author Unknown*

# A Prayer for Baby—Body and Soul

Lord, my baby's bone marrow is completely in charge of making his body's red blood cells now. You do think of everything, don't you? I'm amazed at how you intricately design the parts of the body we'll never even see.

God, I want my child to love you with the deepest part of him, all the way down to his marrow, so to speak. So many people claim to know you, but I want so much more than that for my child. I want him to know you deeply, to have a real and intimate relationship with you. I want him to long for your presence. I want him to crave your word. I want him to ache to hear your voice.

I know I play a huge role in my child's relationship with you—whether it's just on the surface or goes deep down in his heart and soul. Give me a bottomless desire for you, Lord, and help me pass it down to him.

*In Jesus' name, Amen.*

*Before I formed you in the womb I knew you, before you were born I set you apart.* —Jeremiah 1:5a

# Baby's Physical Development

Your baby is getting more cramped in your uterus, but that won't stop his activity. He is starting to regulate his own temperature, and his bone marrow has taken over red blood cell production. His eyelashes are developing, and he's urinating half a liter a day! He weighs about two and a half pounds at this point.

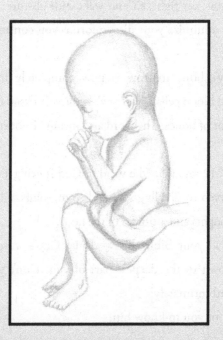

# Mom's Development—Body and Soul

Back pain, leg cramps, shortness of breath—just some of the discomforts of the final weeks of pregnancy. If you're feeling great, revel in it! Few women reach the end of their term feeling very comfortable.

You'll be hearing and reading the same things over and over: get exercise and rest, eat right, sit and walk with posture. All of these tips will help minimize your discomfort as you continue to grow. And grow.

Your baby's bone marrow is now completely in charge of producing red blood cells. "Marrow" is the soft tissue found in the hollow interior of bones. The word also means "inmost or essential part."

Hebrews 4:12 says that "the word of God is living and active . . . it penetrates even to dividing soul and spirit, joints and marrow; it judges the thoughts and attitudes of the heart."

As you read your Bible this week, let God's words penetrate your soul, down to the deepest part of you. Don't you want to know the Lord intimately?

He longs for you to know him.

Before I formed you in the womb I knew you, before you were born I set you apart. —Jeremiah 1:5a

# In Your Words

Describe a time you felt closest to God.

_____

_____

_____

_____

_____

_____

_____

_____

_____

_____

_____

_____

_____

_____

_____

_____

_____

_____

_____

# Inner Beauty ∼Hair

When Elizabeth heard Mary's greeting, the baby leaped in her womb, and Elizabeth was filled with the Holy Spirit. In a loud voice she exclaimed: "Blessed are you among women, and blessed is the child you will bear! . . . As soon as the sound of your greeting reached my ears, the baby in my womb leaped for joy."

*LUKE 1:41–42, 44*

*If your baby is "beautiful and perfect, never cries or fusses, sleeps on schedule and burps on demand, an angel all the time," you're the grandma.*

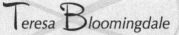

Teresa Bloomingdale

# Mom's Development—Body and Soul

Have you noticed some swelling in your legs and ankles? This is common in late pregnancy, especially when you've been on your feet a lot. If the swelling is rapid, or your hands and feet begin to swell, call your doctor.

Hopefully, the joys of your pregnancy are outweighing the pains. If you're having a rough go of it, counting your blessings—even putting them in writing—will help.

Full-bodied, shiny hair is one thing you can put on that list. And guess what, your little one may have hair by now too! Some babies are born bald, some have tons of hair—you just never know.

Remember, Mama, as you get bigger and bigger, that a beautiful spirit is more important than outward appearances. Pretty is as pretty does, so the saying goes. If you are kind, loving, and sweet to those around you, they'll see beauty no matter what you look like physically. But just so you know, a pregnant woman is a lovely thing to behold.

Be beautiful inside and out this week.

Inner Beauty

# A Prayer for Baby—Body and Soul

Lord, I can't wait to see if my baby has hair or not! Will she be born with peach fuzz, curly tufts, or a head as bald as a bowling ball? Will her hair be dark or light or somewhere in between?

God, thank you for giving us hair. It's just one more thing that adds to our uniqueness. Your hair can say so much about you—your tastes, your style, your creative nature. May my child be content with whatever kind of hair you put on her sweet little head. May she find it uniquely beautiful.

I pray that she will live a long and full life—that someday she'll have gray hair (although she'll probably dye it!). Gray hair is a sign of maturity and wisdom—of age and experience. Help her not to dread getting older, but to embrace the beauty of each year you give her here on earth. Help her to look forward to the day when her time here is done, and you take her home.

*In Jesus' name, Amen.*

*Before I formed you in the womb I knew you, before you were born I set you apart. —Jeremiah 1:5a*

# Baby's Physical Development

Your baby is nearing the three-pound mark. Her eyes may be wide open, though there isn't much for her to see. She is aware of her surroundings, and she can sense light and darkness from outside the womb. She might have hair! Her lungs are still developing during this crucial time.

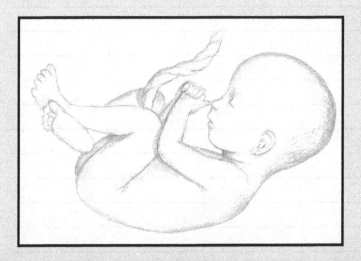

# In Your Words

Make a list of all the ways God made you beautiful.

_____

_____

_____

_____

_____

_____

_____

_____

_____

_____

_____

_____

_____

_____

_____

_____

_____

Before I formed you in the womb I knew you, before you were born I set you apart. —Jeremiah 1:5a

# WEEK 31

## Insight Eyes

*I lift up my eyes to the hills—*
*where does my help come from?*
*My help comes from the LORD,*
*the Maker of heaven and earth.*

PSALM 121:1–2

*How far that little candle throws his beams!*
*So shines a good deed in a weary world.*

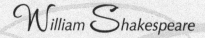
William Shakespeare

# A Prayer for Baby—Body and Soul

Lord, thank you for creating our eyes. Thank you that my baby's eyes are open, that his irises dilate and contract according to how much light is let into my womb. Thank you for designing us so intricately. Our bodies are so adaptable, right down to the tiniest parts.

God, will you give my child eyes that recognize the beauty of the world around him? From a very early age, will you instill in him an understanding that all this beauty was created by someone—and that that someone was you? Give him insight into the nature of his Creator.

Open his eyes to the hidden treasures of this planet. Give him a curiosity about his environment, a love for the earth you created. And when he enjoys the grass and trees and the sky and the sunset, may he praise your holy name and give you all the glory.

Glory to you, Lord, for your miraculous creation!

In Jesus' name, I pray. Amen.

Before I formed you in the womb I knew you, before you were born I set you apart. —Jeremiah 1:5a

# Baby's Physical Development

Your baby weighs about three pounds, five ounces now. He's around fifteen and a half inches long. He can track moving objects with his eyes, and his irises dilate and contract. His lungs and digestive tract are just about mature. He swallows amniotic fluid and urinates several cups of fluid per day.

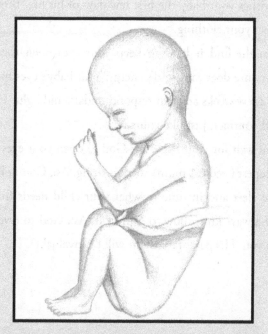

# Mom's Development—Body and Soul

Are you ready for your baby to be born yet? Your "weeks to go" countdown is in single digits now. Baby still has a lot of growing to do, so everything will keep getting bigger and tighter.

Don't be alarmed if your breasts start leaking. Around this time, your milk glands start producing colostrum—the premilk that nourishes your baby the first few days of his life. Breast pads will protect your clothing.

You might find it hard to keep your eyes open these days. Pregnancy sure does zap a girl's energy. Your baby's eyes have been open for a few weeks and can respond to dark and light. His irises dilate and contract, just like yours do.

As you wait for your baby, ask God to open your eyes to your child's deepest needs. A mom's work is tiring. Ask God to help you always be alert and in tune to what your child needs from you. He won't always know how to express it. Ask God to reveal these things to you. His parental insight will be invaluable.

*Before I formed you in the womb I knew you, before you were born I set you apart. —Jeremiah 1:5a*

# In Your Words

Go outside or look out a window, and describe the beauty you see.
What insights does it give you into the mind and heart of your
Creator?

_____

_____

_____

_____

_____

_____

_____

_____

_____

_____

_____

_____

_____

_____

_____

_____

_____

_____

# WEEK 32
## Strength ∽ Muscles

The LORD gives strength to his people;
the LORD blesses his people with peace.

*PSALM 29:11*

*The strength of a man consists in finding out the way
God is going, and going that way.*

Henry Ward Beecher

# Mom's Development—Body and Soul

Did you tell yourself when you first got pregnant that you wouldn't be one of those "waddling" pregnant women? How's that plan working out for you? Pregnancy hormones have relaxed your joints, and you really are moving differently. Your center of gravity has also shifted dramatically. There are different degrees of waddle, but you probably won't be able to avoid it altogether.

Exercise will help keep your muscles in the best shape possible. And your little baby's muscles are going through a growth spurt right about now! The weight she's putting on is largely due to the increase in muscle tissue.

You may not feel like you have a lot of strength right now. What a perfect time to rely on God! Ask him this week to give you a generous outpouring of his strength. The Bible is full of verses that speak to God's strength being sufficient when we ourselves are weak. Look up some of them in the next couple days.

You can do all things through Christ who gives you strength!

Strength

157

# A Prayer for Baby—Body and Soul

Father, my baby has been gaining lots of muscle lately. She's getting stronger and stronger with each passing day. Lord, I want my child to be strong—not just physically, but emotionally, mentally, and spiritually.

I pray that you will give her the strength to always stand up for what is right. I think especially of her teenage years when negative peer pressure will be a real and frightening force. God, help her to stand firm in you. Give her the strength to resist any temptation that goes against your word. Help her to stand strong and fast in the midst of adversity.

Give her the confidence that she can do anything you ask her to do. Remind her of Philippians 4:13—"I can do everything through him who gives me strength."

Help me to build a foundation of truth into her life at a young age, so she'll have the tools she needs to be strong.

I praise you, my strong and almighty God.

In Jesus' name, Amen.

Before I formed you in the womb I knew you, before you were born I set you apart. —*Jeremiah 1:5a*

# Baby's Physical Development

Your baby weighs close to four pounds now. As her fat and muscle tissue continue to develop, she'll keep rapidly gaining weight. The fine lanugo is being shed from her body, and she's growing eyelashes, eyebrows, and hair. She's running out of space in your womb!

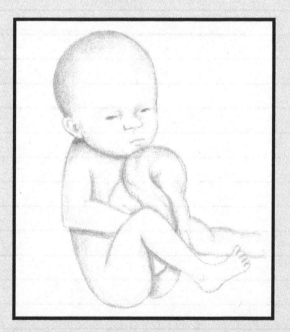

Strength

# In Your Words

Look up (and write down) some Bible verses about the Lord being
your strength.

_____

_____

_____

_____

_____

_____

_____

_____

_____

_____

_____

_____

_____

_____

*Before I formed you in the womb I knew you,
before you were born I set you apart. —Jeremiah 1:5a*

# WEEK 33

# Sexual Purity ∽ Testicles

So in the course of time Hannah
conceived and gave birth to a son.
She named him Samuel, saying,
"Because I asked the LORD for him."

*1 SAMUEL 1:20*

*What are little boys made of?*
*What are little boys made of?*
*Frogs and snails and puppy-dog tails,*
*That's what little boys are made of.*

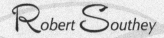

Robert Southey

# A Prayer for Baby—Body and Soul

Father, thank you for the little baby growing inside my womb. If I'm carrying a boy, this is a big week for him. His testicles are descending into his scrotum from inside his body where you formed and fashioned them. I don't pretend to have any idea how you create our bodies with the capacity for reproduction. What evidence for a Creator!

Lord, I pray for sexual purity for my son. He's being born into a world that has cheapened sex. You created it as a pure and precious gift for him to share with his wife someday, and our culture has twisted and abused it. I know it's going to take a lifetime of prayer and wisdom on my part to help him stay pure. Will you fill his heart with a desire to honor you with his actions?

And God, I pray that you will bless him with the ability to father children. I want him to experience the joy and amazement of parenthood.

In Jesus' name, Amen.

Before I formed you in the womb I knew you, before you were born I set you apart. —Jeremiah 1:5a

# Baby's Physical Development

Your baby weighs around four and a half pounds now and is rapidly putting on weight—mostly in the form of fat. There are billions of neurons in his brain, allowing him to hear, feel, and see. His testicles are descending into his scrotum, and his lungs have nearly matured. You might have noticed him hiccupping in utero.

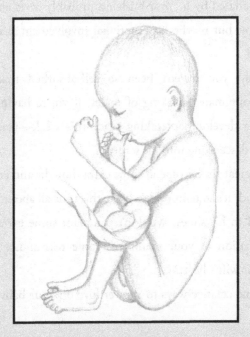

# Mom's Development—Body and Soul

Baby's father hasn't gotten much attention so far in this book, has he? Of course, it was written for you, and you're the one carrying the baby, but Dad is important too. How is he dealing with your pregnancy and the impending birth of his child?

Some men love the whole pregnancy experience. Others are pretty intimidated by it. Your husband probably cares about you and the baby, but maybe his emotional involvement is less than you'd hoped.

Hopefully, you haven't been so self-absorbed that you've neglected your man. Speaking of males, if you're having a boy, there's a big development taking place this week—your baby's testicles are descending into his scrotum.

What a great time to spend some extra thought and energy on your husband. It's so tempting to make this time all about you, but put yourself in his shoes. Wouldn't you want some extra loving, some affirmation of your manhood, some reassurance of your place in your wife's heart?

Find some creative ways to shower love on your baby's daddy this week.

*Before I formed you in the womb I knew you, before you were born I set you apart.* —Jeremiah 1:5a

# In Your Words

Make a list of everything you love about your husband. Then share it with him.

_____

_____

_____

_____

_____

_____

_____

_____

_____

_____

_____

_____

_____

_____

_____

_____

_____

_____

_____

_____

_____

# Conviction ❧ Skeleton

Stand firm then, with the belt of truth
buckled around your waist,
with the breastplate of righteousness
in place, and with your feet fitted
with the readiness that comes
from the gospel of peace.

*EPHESIANS 6:14–15*

There are two lasting bequests we can give our
children. One is roots. The other is wings.

Hodding Carter, Jr.

# Mom's Development—Body and Soul

Are all your plans coming together? Are you ready for this little baby's arrival? You probably know people who have had their babies a few weeks early. Do you ever wonder if you might be one of them? It's not very likely, but your baby really could come at any time.

Rest is good. Are you getting enough? Are you taking time to put up your feet, breathe deeply, and do absolutely nothing? Take advantage of these final weeks before Baby arrives on the scene.

And drink lots of milk! Or find some way to get plenty of calcium. Your baby's skeleton is hardening, and she needs calcium to make those bones hard and strong. You'll want to stay strong too—and not just physically.

As you think about your baby's skeleton firming up, think about the things you stand firm for—your personal values and convictions. Ask God for strength to stay true to him and his word—to stand strong when your faith is questioned. And it will be.

Conviction

# A Prayer for Baby—Body and Soul

Lord, I want my little one to be physically strong. As I think about her frame, I pray that she'll be a sturdy little thing. Harden those bones, so she'll be able to withstand the bumps and knocks of life. I don't want her to be fragile or easily broken. I pray that she will be able to stand straight and tall all the days of her life.

And may she stand tall for truth and righteousness as well. When those around her are unsure of their beliefs, when their convictions crumble, may she stand firm and fast. Help me to instill in her a knowledge of the truth. May she be so familiar with your truth that she can recognize a lie from a mile away. Lord, don't let her be dragged down by deceptive philosophies the world is so quick to offer.

Make her strong. Thank you for being her strong tower. She can run to you, lean on you, and you'll never fail her.

Bless your name, Lord.

*In Jesus' name, Amen.*

*Before I formed you in the womb I knew you, before you were born I set you apart.* —Jeremiah 1:5a

# Baby's Physical Development

Your baby weighs about five pounds now and could easily thrive outside your womb. Her lungs are fairly well developed, and she is most likely in the head-down position. The vernix coating is thickening and the lanugo hair is disappearing. Her skeleton is hardening, so she needs her mother to take in plenty of calcium.

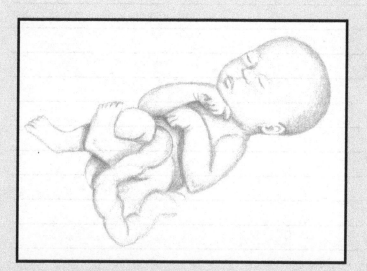

*Conviction*

# In Your Words

What are some core beliefs of your faith?

_____

_____

_____

_____

_____

_____

_____

_____

_____

_____

_____

_____

_____

_____

_____

_____

_____

_____

Before I formed you in the womb I knew you,
before you were born I set you apart. —Jeremiah 1:5a

## Praise ∽ Lungs

> From birth I have relied on you; you
> brought me forth from my mother's womb.
> I will ever praise you.
>
> PSALM 71:6

*Were there no God, we would be in this glorious*
*world with grateful hearts and no one to thank.*

Christina Rossetti

# A Prayer for Baby—Body and Soul

Lord, I can't tell you how thankful I am that my baby's lungs are finally in perfect working order. I feel like I can breathe so much more easily now knowing he'd be just fine if he came early. Please continue to strengthen those little lungs in these last few weeks.

I pray that my child will use his lungs for your glory—to sing and shout praises to you, God. I love the book of Psalms. I love how the psalmist expresses his love and awe for you through singing and shouting. I pray that my child will long to worship you, not just in his heart, but out loud with songs of praise.

It doesn't matter if he can carry a tune. It doesn't matter if he was blessed with rhythm. You see right through us, to our hearts, and you're glorified when we express our adoration in an outward, physical way.

My heart thrills at the thought of worshiping you alongside my child—together praising our Savior.

In Jesus' name, Amen.

Before I formed you in the womb I knew you, before you were born I set you apart. —Jeremiah 1:5a

# Baby's Physical Development

Your baby weighs over five pounds now and is gaining about half a pound each week. Remember, this is only an average. Full-term babies can weigh anywhere from five to ten pounds—or more. There isn't much room for your baby to move around, so he may punch and kick less often, but he'll do it with greater force. His lungs are finally fully developed!

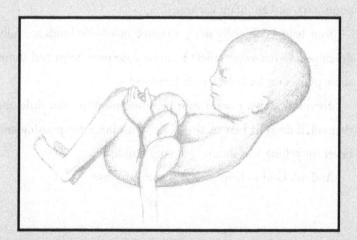

# Mom's Development—Body and Soul

Are you a planner? Is your hospital bag packed? No one likes the thought of her water breaking at the grocery store and being unprepared. You've probably read all kinds of books and articles telling you what to take to the hospital.

Some of the most important things? For you: a cozy pillow, socks, slippers, soap, shampoo, a camera, a pen and journal, and a comfy outfit that you wore when you were five months pregnant (really!). For Baby: his baby book, a going-home outfit in two sizes (there's a big difference between five-pound babies and nine-pounders), and an infant car seat.

Your baby is officially ready to come now—his lungs are fully developed. What sweet relief! Exercise your own lungs and shout some praises to the Lord for his goodness.

Then lean down toward your belly and promise your little one that you'll do your best to always use your lungs for praising and never for yelling and shouting at your child.

And ask God to help you keep your promise.

*Before I formed you in the womb I knew you, before you were born I set you apart. —Jeremiah 1:5a*

# In Your Words

Write a simple song of praise to the Lord (or copy one from the Psalms), and then sing it to him.

_____

_____

_____

_____

_____

_____

_____

_____

_____

_____

_____

_____

_____

_____

_____

_____

_____

# WEEK 36
## Work Ethic ∽ Sweat

May the favor of the Lord our God rest upon us; establish the work of our hands for us—yes, establish the work of our hands.

PSALM 90:17

*Be strong! We are not here to play, to dream, to drift;*
*We have hard work to do and loads to lift;*
*Shun not the struggle—face it; 'tis God's gift.*

## Maltbie D. Babcock

# Mom's Development—Body and Soul

Your last month of pregnancy! Can you believe it? It's time to start seeing your practitioner every week. You'll be checked for fun stats like effacement and dilation. Don't get discouraged if you don't see much "progress." Babies pay little attention to these measures and come when they're ready.

Having trouble sleeping? Peeing every five minutes? Feeling big and uncomfortable? It won't be long now. Try your best to relax and enjoy these last few weeks.

Can you believe your baby is sweating in utero and has been for several weeks? Hopefully you're able to take it easy and aren't sweating from overexertion. There will be plenty of time for hard work and getting things accomplished. Right now, you just focus on growing that baby.

After she's born, and you're plenty rested, you can get back to the hard work you're used to doing. And be sure to view your work—especially mundane chores like dishes and diaper changing—as an act of worship, because it is. You can glorify God in every single thing you do, no matter how simple or common.

Work Ethic

# A Prayer for Baby—Body and Soul

Lord, I thank you for all of my baby's bodily functions—even sweating. It's amazing how you created our bodies to regulate themselves and do so much on their own. Thank you for sweat that cools down our bodies so we don't overheat.

I pray that you will bless my child's hard work as she grows. Help her to see the value in hard work. Help me to model a strong work ethic, not laziness. Help her to set about her chores with a willing spirit and view them as a way to give back to you.

Will you establish the work of her hands, Father? There is so much satisfaction in a job well done. And it can be such a disappointment when hard work is wasted. May her work be profitable and may she enjoy the fruits of her labor.

Thank you for allowing us the privilege to work and to find joy in what we do. May her work be fulfilling in every way.

In Jesus' name, Amen.

Before I formed you in the womb I knew you, before you were born I set you apart. —Jeremiah 1:5a

# Baby's Physical Development

Your baby probably weighs close to six pounds at this point. There is meat on her little bones, and she's even starting to sweat! The bones of her skull haven't fused together yet. They are capable of overlapping, allowing the baby to fit through the birth canal. If your baby's head is cone shaped, don't worry. It will round out soon enough.

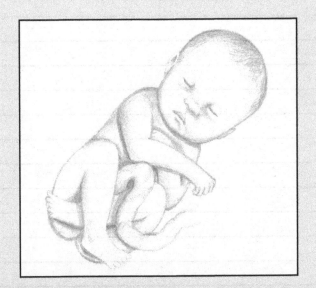

Work Ethic

# In Your Words

Think of your least favorite tasks (chores, errands, etc.). How might you go about them in a way that brings glory to God?

_____

_____

_____

_____

_____

_____

_____

_____

_____

_____

_____

_____

_____

_____

_____

_____

*Before I formed you in the womb I knew you, before you were born I set you apart.* —Jeremiah 1:5a

# Anticipation ✑ Fingers

> *Yet this I call to mind and therefore I have hope: Because of the Lord's great love we are not consumed, for his compassions never fail. They are new every morning; great is your faithfulness.*
>
> *LAMENTATIONS 3:21–23*

*One of the most powerful handclasps is that of a new grandbaby around the finger of a grandfather.*

*Joy Hargrove*

# A Prayer for Baby—Body and Soul

Father, thank you for my baby's ten little fingers and ten tiny toes. I can't believe he can grasp already. I know one thing: he already has me wrapped around one of his miniature fingers!

God, I can't wait for my baby to touch me with his hands, to curl his fingers around one of mine. What an unspeakable blessing!

Will you help him as he grows to always grasp tightly the important things in life? I want him to know that life isn't about money and possessions or success and awards. I want him to hold tightly to God and family, to loving and serving others, to making a difference in his world that will last into eternity.

I want him to look forward to each new day with excitement and anticipation. I hope he wakes up wondering, "What does God have in store for me today?"

As long as my child holds tight to you, his can be a life of unparalleled adventure.

In Jesus' name, Amen.

Before I formed you in the womb I knew you, before you were born I set you apart. —Jeremiah 1:5a

# Baby's Physical Development

Your baby probably weighs somewhere in the neighborhood of six pounds now. At the end of this week, he'll be considered full-term. He has enough fat to keep him warm outside your womb and will keep adding fat until birth. He is coordinated enough now to grasp with his fingers.

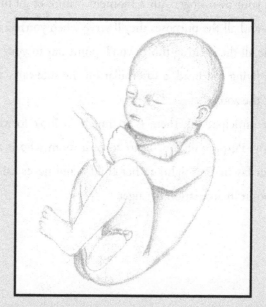

# Mom's Development—Body and Soul

You're getting so close, girl! In just a matter of days, you'll have a baby in your arms! Aren't you just so excited to finally meet your little one?

Your baby is learning new tricks all the time. He is now coordinated enough to grasp things with his fingers. Who knows? Maybe he's busy playing tug-of-war with the umbilical cord.

Look at your own fingers for a moment. Think of all the uses they have—and all the purposes they'll serve when you're a mom. Just imagine all the exciting things you'll point out to your child: an airplane flying overhead, a caterpillar on the sidewalk, a baby flamingo at the zoo. . . .

Oh, the anticipation! There is so much to look forward to as a mommy! Purpose in your heart to be a mom who is always pointing out fascinating sights to her child—and never using her fingers to point in accusation or anger.

*Before I formed you in the womb I knew you, before you were born I set you apart. —Jeremiah 1:5a*

# In Your Words

Imagine all the wonderful sights you'll be able to see through your child's eyes. Make a list of the things you're most excited to show him.

_____

_____

_____

_____

_____

_____

_____

_____

_____

_____

_____

_____

_____

_____

_____

_____

_____

_____

_____

Anticipation

# Comfort ∾ Arms

Praise be to the God and Father of our Lord Jesus Christ, the Father of compassion and the God of all comfort, who comforts us in all our troubles, so that we can comfort those in any trouble with the comfort we ourselves have received from God.

2 CORINTHIANS 1:3–4

*I remember my mother's prayers,
and they have always followed me.
They have clung to me all my life.*

Abraham Lincoln

# Mom's Development—Body and Soul

Your baby is officially considered full-term now! Be sure to let her know she's welcome to come at any time. A due date doesn't mean much—only 5 percent of babies are born on that day.

As uncomfortable—even miserable—as you may be, try to soak up these last few weeks of pregnancy. You might be surprised to find out how much you miss having your baby squirming around inside of you.

Your little one is able to flex her arms now. Her muscles aren't bulging, of course, but they're getting stronger the more she uses them. Your own arms are about to get a workout. Your newborn won't weigh much, but as you hold, carry, rock, burp, and feed her, you'll use muscles you didn't know you had.

There are few things on earth more comforting than a mother's arms. Pray this week that God will help you always keep your arms wide open to your child. May your embrace be a calm, safe place for her to run to.

Comfort

# A Prayer for Baby—Body and Soul

Father, thank you for my baby's arms. She can flex her tiny muscles now. They're developed enough to tighten up and relax. As she punches me from the inside out, I can tell she's busy putting those new muscles to good use!

God, I pray that she will use her arms to reach out to others, to be an encouragement and a comfort to those in need. There's just something about a hug that can brighten a day, soothe a broken heart, even save a life.

Help me to be an example to her of nurture and comfort. May she always remember feeling safe and loved in her mama's arms. Someday when she has a family of her own, may she lovingly wrap her arms around them every chance she gets.

I pray that she will always use her arms in a way that brings glory to you.

In Jesus' name, Amen.

Before I formed you in the womb I knew you, before you were born I set you apart. —Jeremiah 1:5a

# Baby's Physical Development

Your baby could weigh anywhere from six to eight pounds or more at this point. If she were born today, she'd be perfectly formed and ready to go. She can grasp things very firmly now and can even flex her arm muscles. She's losing her vernix coating, although many newborns are born with it in their skin creases and folds.

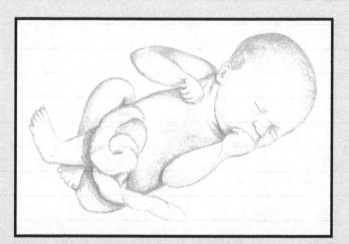

Comfort

# In Your Words

Do you remember what it felt like to be wrapped in the comfort of your mother's (or grandmother's) arms? Describe that feeling.

_____

_____

_____

_____

_____

_____

_____

_____

_____

_____

_____

_____

_____

_____

_____

_____

*Before I formed you in the womb I knew you, before you were born I set you apart. —Jeremiah 1:5a*

# Creative Force ∽ Organs

> As you do not know the path of the wind,
> or how the body is formed in a mother's
> womb, so you cannot understand the work
> of God, the Maker of all things.
>
> *ECCLESIASTES 11:5*

*Every child is an artist. The problem is how to remain an artist once he grows up.*

# Pablo Picasso

# A Prayer for Baby—Body and Soul

Father, thank you that my baby's organs are now all completely developed and ready to function perfectly outside the comforts of his mama's body. I will never know how you did it—and on such a tight schedule! Ingenious! You crafted everything so beautifully, and your timing is so perfect. Thank you!

I pray for the health of my baby. Will you bring him safely into this world? I pray that his heart is beating strongly, his lungs working correctly, his digestive system functioning smoothly.

And God, will you continue to protect him as he grows? You fashioned him from the beginning, and you, our great Physician, can heal him from any sickness or disease. You created us and know exactly how to fix us. I praise you for that, Lord!

I stand in awe of you, my Creator God.

*In Jesus' name, Amen.*

*Before I formed you in the womb I knew you, before you were born I set you apart. —Jeremiah 1:5a*

# Baby's Physical Development

Your baby probably weighs at least six pounds and could weigh a lot more. His fingernails are getting longer. His lanugo is gone. His organs are developed. He has defined tissue in his chest. He has mastered several reflexes, including grasping, sucking, and flexing. He's feeling confined, and he wants out!

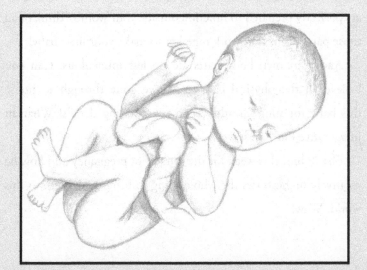

# Mom's Development—Body and Soul

Ooooh, there's excitement (and anxiety and apprehension) in the air! Your baby will be here soon! Have you felt the "nesting" instinct yet? Some women describe this as an overwhelming urge to get things clean (spotless!), organized, and ready for Baby's arrival. About-to-pop pregnant gals have been known to dust every baseboard in the house, stock up on a year's worth of toilet paper, or scrub the bathtub with their husband's toothbrush.

Your baby will come when he's good and ready. All his organs are perfectly prepared to function outside your womb. Think of all those parts of his that work together to make your little baby!

And your own body parts are no less miraculous. Can you believe all the physical changes you've gone through to house this baby for nine months? So many amazing details! What an imaginative God we serve!

Thank him this week for the miracle of pregnancy and how he creatively orchestrates the whole thing to bring new life into this world. Wow!

*Before I formed you in the womb I knew you, before you were born I set you apart. —Jeremiah 1:5a*

# In Your Words

What body parts or functions are the most amazing to you? Describe your awe, then thank God for his creative genius.

_____

_____

_____

_____

_____

_____

_____

_____

_____

_____

_____

_____

_____

_____

_____

_____

_____

_____

# WEEK 40
## Joy ∽ First Cry

A woman giving birth to a child has
pain because her time has come; but when
her baby is born she forgets the anguish
because of her joy that a child is
born into the world.

*JOHN 16:21*

*The moment a child is born, the mother
is also born. She never existed before.
The woman existed, but the mother, never.
A mother is something absolutely new.*

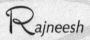

Rajneesh

# Mom's Development—Body and Soul

Are you sad to see this book end? This journey has been so much fun! But you're starting a new chapter in your life now.

One of these days you'll look back at your pregnancy and think, "Wow, that seems like a lifetime ago." Thankfully, you have mementos like this one to help you recall your precious memories of this oh-so-special time.

Imagine hearing your baby's first cry—the one thing she couldn't do in the womb. The sound of that cry will bring a wave of relief and joy washing over you like nothing you've ever felt in your life. Your baby is here. She's finally here. And she's okay.

She probably won't be the only one crying. There will be tears of joy in your eyes and your hubby's, and in the eyes of the slew of family members who come to visit in the days ahead. When you get a moment, cry out to God on behalf of your priceless child. Share your mother-joy with your heavenly Father.

Ask him to bless and keep your little one every moment of her life.

# A Prayer for Baby—Body and Soul

Oh, Father, my baby will be here any day now. I can hardly wait to meet her. Oh, I pray she lets out a wail that rings through the hospital halls. I want her to announce her presence with gusto: "I'm here, world! Here I am!"

I'm sure I'll change my tune soon enough—when it's the middle of the night and I can't get her to stop crying—but for now, I want to hear those lungs fill with air and that cry to echo off the walls.

Dear Lord, as my child grows, will you fill her little heart to overflowing? I long to hear her crying out in joy to her Lord and Savior. You are the only one who can ultimately meet her every need and desire. Help me to show her from an early age that you will never fail her and that you are the one true source of joy.

Thank you for this precious child, God.

In Jesus' name, Amen.

Before I formed you in the womb I knew you, before you were born I set you apart. —Jeremiah 1:5a

# Baby's Physical Development

Your baby is ready for her big day! She's big enough, strong enough, and eager enough to come on out and join the party. Think of all the sensations she'll experience for the first time: the cool air, the feel of a blanket, human contact, loud noises, pain, hunger—even her first audible cry. Hold her tight, love her like crazy, and tell her how happy you are that she's yours.

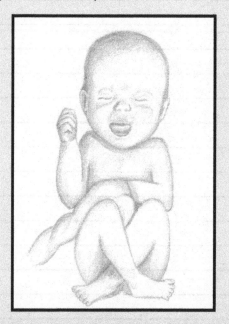

# In Your Words

Write a joyful heart-prayer to God for your precious little child.

_____

_____

_____

_____

_____

_____

_____

_____

_____

_____

_____

_____

_____

_____

_____

_____

*Before I formed you in the womb I knew you, before you were born I set you apart. —Jeremiah 1:5a*

# About the Author

Marla Taviano is the author of *Is That All He Thinks About?*, *Changing Your World One Diaper at a Time*, *The Husband's Guide to Getting Lucky*, *Once Upon the Internet*, *The Wife Life*, *We Dream of Cambodia*, *An Unschooling Manifesto*, and *The Storm*.

Through the generosity of her friends and blog readers, hundreds of copies of her book *Expecting* have been donated to crisis pregnancy centers around the world.

In her former life, Marla was a professional speaker on topics such as sex and parenting but, ever since a trip to Cambodia in 2010, her biggest passion has been loving the poor, seeking justice, and sharing the hope of the gospel.

In January 2015, she and her family moved to Cambodia to work with the Hard Places Community, where they run a drop-in center for at-risk kiddos who live near the world-famous temple Angkor Wat. They work to restore kids who have been sexually abused and exploited and seek to prevent it from happening to others.

Marla and her husband, Gabe, live in a house right next to the center with their awesome, unschooled daughters—Olivia (15), Ava (13), and Nina (10).

It's not an easy life, but it's a beautiful one.